COUNSELING THE COMMUNICATIVELY DISORDERED AND THEIR FAMILIES

COUNSELING THE COMMUNICATIVELY DISORDERED AND THEIR FAMILIES

DAVID LUTERMAN, D. Ed.
Professor of Communication Disorders and Director,
Thayer Lindsley Nursery, Robbins Speech and Hearing Center,
Emerson College, Boston, Massachusetts

Foreword by Alvin J. Davis
Director, Constance Brown Hearing and Speech Center,
Kalamazoo, Michigan

Little, Brown and Company
Boston/Toronto

To Gene McDonald, a mentor

CONTENTS

FOREWORD

In a rather fundamental way, this book is about friendship. It is about becoming and being a friend, to self and to others. This is a very personal book, something of a reflective memoir. Much more than most, this is a philosophical book: it has a clear point of view. You will have no difficulty recognizing David Luterman's feeling, responsive, human center.

For more than 25 years, David Luterman has been for me a loving, sharing, helpful, and growth-provoking friend. Since we shared our professional beginnings as graduate students in speech pathology and audiology at Penn State, I have known David to be a "people person." From the privileged perspective of a good and long-time friend, I take great joy in introducing this wise and much-needed text to all who would be a friend to those who struggle with a communication disorder.

Alvin J. Davis

PREFACE

More than 20 years ago I started my career as a clinical audiologist. At that time I thought I was interested in the precision and surety that working with machines seemed to give. I soon realized that I was not a "machine person" but rather a "people person" and that the audiologic machinery was getting in the way of my relating to people. It was with some trepidation that I decided to come out from behind my audiometer and relate as a person rather than as a professional. The first outward manifestation of my slowly evolving inner changes was the willingness to wear nonwhite shirts; soon I went tieless. A few years later, I abandoned suits and sports jackets—the uniform of the male professional. Most recently I have given up all titles and prefer people to call me by my first name. These changes took more than 10 years to accomplish.

Rather than make a radical change in my life, I sought another way of relating to the hearing-impaired population. It became apparent to me that parents of severely hearing-impaired children were not being treated well. I was the clinical audiologist who confirmed the parents' suspicion that they had a deaf child, who then proceeded to talk extensively about a course of action, and who then referred them to an educational facility. My information-giving was designed to keep me in control of the situation, to conform to the parents' expectations and my own perception of what a professional was, and to distance the parents from their feelings, which I did not know how to handle. It also became apparent to me, on subsequent visits, that the needs of parents were not being met by either the educational facilities or myself. So with a great deal of naiveté, I decided in 1965 to begin a parent-centered nursery program at Emerson College in Boston. In addition to a nursery and language therapy, the Emerson program provided a once-a-week session designed as a parent support group, which I led. I decided early to forego my information-providing function (I had to—I had only a small number of set speeches and I was committing myself to 30 sessions with the parents) and spent much of each session listening to the parents. The program has continued to the present and has afforded me a great opportunity to grow both personally and professionally. Out of my experience came a book describing the program in detail with procedures for counseling parents of hearing-impaired children (Luterman, 1979).

I found as I allowed more affect (feelings) to enter into these relationships (I could, for example, allow the parents to cry), listened more, and dealt less with content, that people learned more. When the information was spaced over time, and when I allowed parents to work through their very normal feelings about having a deaf child, the parents could absorb and retain the information I was providing. I realized that all those brilliant set speeches that I had been delivering had not been retained by the parents anyway, as on subsequent visits I found that parents were asking me questions that I thought I had already covered adequately. I also discovered that people were not as fragile as I had thought (actually, it was my own fragility I had been worrying about) and that they could defend themselves quite well against my insensitivities and all-too-frequent lack of skill. As long as I remained a caring, listening person, growth occurred within the relationship. I seemed to serve parents much better when I did not function in the traditional information-providing mode. As an added bonus I found that my professional boredom was replaced by excitement.

During the past several years, I have been teaching courses and giving workshops on counseling issues to working audiologists and speech pathologists. These experiences have made me aware that attitudes have not changed very much regarding counseling in the 20-odd years since I started working as a professional. Counseling as practiced by most audiologists and speech-language pathologists still seems to be of the information-imparting or advice-giving variety (i.e., the medical or quasi-medical model). If the relationship between the professional and the individual with communication disorders gets into the emotional area, the audiologist/speech-language pathologist becomes uncomfortable and tends to hide behind content or to refer the patient to a social worker or psychologist. The information-providing role, however, is not satisfactory over the long run. One is apt to get bored delivering all the set speeches accumulated over a working lifetime. Professionals dealing with communication disorders who wish to change tend, after a few years of information-providing, to seek other ways of relating to those they are servicing; hence the attendance at workshops on counseling.

Those professionals who do not find another way of relating tend to "burn out" quickly. The burnout rate in our field is quite high; 43 percent of surveyed speech pathologists reported moderate to severe burnout, which involved a loss of concern for the feelings of their client (Miller and Potter, 1982).

I think it is generally acknowledged that counseling skills are an important concomitant of the well-trained speech pathologist, yet little formal training is provided in educational programs. An examination of graduate catalogs indicates few courses offered specifically on counseling for the speech clinician, nor is a course in counseling required for certification by the American Speech-Language-Hearing Association. Counseling skills, when they are obtained by graduate clinicians, seem to be obtained informally through students' observation of other clinicians or almost incidentally picked up as students acquire specific skills in altering speech and language behavior. Too many of our students are leaving training programs with a very limited view of their capacity to involve themselves in intensive relationships with their clients.

This book was initiated—as I suspect many texts are—when I agreed to teach a course on counseling the communicatively disordered and found that there was no single, satisfactory text. The ultimate purpose of this book is to demystify the counseling experience for the professional working within the field of communication disorders. It is my hope that as a result of reading this book, clinicians will feel more comfortable in allowing the affect that is a normal concomitant of having a communication disorder to emerge in their clinical interactions. I hope this book will provide some insight into relationship-building and how it affects the counseling process. By allowing more affect to occur in the relationships, speech-language pathologists and audiologists will find that their information-providing role will be enhanced and they will therefore be much more effective. I think they will also obtain more job satisfaction.

This text is not intended to supplant the clinical use of social workers or psychologists: they are trained professionals whose skills will be needed within a comprehensive speech-language and hearing program. I hope, however, that this text will lead to a modified use of professional counselors so that they can provide support and ongoing inservice training to speech pathologists/audiologists as they deal with the normal emotions surrounding a communication disorder and provide direct service to emotionally disordered clients who may also have a communication disorder.

During the past several years I have come to value highly the use of Erik Erikson's stages of growth as a means of understanding both the difficulties of the communicatively disordered and the development of a counseling relationship. Recently I have come across the writings of Irvin Yalom on existential issues in psychotherapy, which I believe have far-reaching implications for the field of communication disorders. This text reflects my expanded appreciation of both Yalom and Erikson.

I have devoted a chapter to group counseling, as I feel that this area of counseling can be better utilized by the speech and hearing clinician. I have also devoted more space to the denial mechanism than I did in my previous book because I have come to see more clearly how the difficulties of the professional in handling the complex issue of denial limits effective counseling.

In writing this book I have drawn heavily on my own experience in the field of deafness and, in particular, on my work with parents. I have made no attempt to delineate content counseling for the specific speech disorders as I assume that the well-trained speech-language pathologist has this information. Once the professional acquires counseling skills, they are applicable to all disorders. By extension, much of the material is also appropriate for other disabling conditions, which do not necessarily involve a communication disorder. I hope that this book is of use to any professional working with the communicatively disordered who wishes to get beyond the information-providing role.

D. L.

BIBLIOGRAPHY

Luterman, D. *Counseling Parents of Hearing-Impaired Children.* Boston: Little, Brown, 1979.

Miller, M., and Potter, R. Professional burnout among speech-language pathologists. *ASHA* 24:177, 1982.

ACKNOWLEDGMENTS

A book, even when it has a single author on its title page as this one does, is really the collaboration of many people. I certainly had a great deal of help in putting this volume together. I wish to thank my friends and colleagues who so generously gave of their time to read and comment on various chapters as I wrote them. Among the many were Judy Chasin, Mary Holdgrafer, Susan Colten, David Maxwell, Jackie Liebergot, Mark Ross, Debbie Cain, and Anita Small. There is probably no more helpful species of professional than a librarian. I had two such helpful ones in Cynthia Alcorn and Mina Rakhra. I often felt they would gladly go to the moon to get me some obscure reference if I needed it. Lisa Alberti had the unenviable task of trying to translate my illegible handwriting to a typed manuscript. She did this with patience and good humor. Part of the proceeds of this book will go to pay for an ophthalmologic examination to see if anything can be done about the squint she has developed. Linda Dolmatch also typed the manuscript, seemingly able to read my mind, and functioned as a careful editor and supporter.

I am grateful to the crew in Edmonton who really got me started on this book. I wish also to acknowledge the support of my children James, Emily, Daniel, and Alison, who had to put up with a very distracted father and who love to see their names in print. My wife Cari provided immense amounts of support, doing innumerable things for me during the writing of this book—I owe her much.

COUNSELING THE COMMUNICATIVELY DISORDERED AND THEIR FAMILIES

A Matter of Pronouns. The problem of pronouns poses a formidable dilemma for the writer at this stage of our social consciousness. I find the construct his/her unbearably awkward. In this volume I have decided to alternate masculine and feminine pronouns by chapter, beginning with feminine in Chapter 1. I hope this will not be confusing to the reader. I look forward to the development of neuter singular pronouns.

CHAPTER 1

COUNSELING AND THE

SPEECH THERAPIST/

AUDIOLOGIST

Counseling is a term that seems to mean many different things to different people. Professional approaches to counseling involve a wide range of behaviors including direct environmental manipulation, advice-giving, persuasion, confrontation, generation of insight, and providing a warm, accepting relationship with the client.

In the profession of speech pathology and audiology, counseling frequently seems to mean information-providing and advice-giving; for example, the audiologist "counsels" the patient regarding hearing aid use and the speech therapist "counsels" after administering a diagnostic evaluation. To what extent the speech and hearing professional can move into the emotional area of counseling is rather undefined—and at issue—in our field. Perkins (1977) thinks it is best that the speech therapist steer a middle course between changing speech behavior and being involved in all areas of a client's life. He believes, however, that it is difficult, if not impossible, to isolate the communication problems from life problems but cautions that psychotherapy is beyond the scope of the clinician. Webster (1966) and Clark (1982), on the other hand, argue strongly for the speech therapist and audiologist to be involved with parents and with the affect that surrounds having a handicapped child. Tanner (1980) points out that the speech pathologist often deals with terminally or catastrophically ill patients and must be sensitive to the affect surrounding the grief reaction.

Blanchard (1982) reports that, after the surgeon, speech-language pathologists are the professionals with the most pre- and postoperative contacts with patients having a laryngectomy. He found that the counseling was often inadequate to meet the needs of the individual. Panbacker (1977) found a similar result with the families of children with cleft palate undergoing surgery. While some onus for inadequate counseling must fall on the surgeon, the speech-language pathologist still must take responsibility for poor counseling about the effects of surgery on speech. What makes these two studies so distressing is that the authors cite earlier studies that also indict inadequate counseling, and the situation does not appear to be improving.

For the purpose of this book, *counseling* is defined as an educative experience occurring between people, which is problem-centered and allows for the expression of feeling (affect), permitting and encouraging growth in both parties. This definition reflects my strong biases regarding counseling and the role of the speech therapist/audiologist in that process. For me, counseling is more than information exchange and more than advice-giving, although these elements may be present. Feelings are a large part of the communication process; when communication is defective, affect tends to be high. It is also my strongly held conviction that, in order for a speech-language pathologist and audiologist to be effective, she will have to address these affective issues. Lee Edward Travis (1957), one of the founders of our field, wrote more than 25 years ago that:

> In years to come, it appears reasonable to suppose that speech pathologists will not only apply successfully the principles and practices of psychotherapy to their specialty but will contribute to the advancement of that which they now borrow from. This supposition would seem to be almost self evident, since speech workers are dealing entirely with problems of communication which is the matrix of psychotherapy (p. 965).

I am not sure that Travis's prediction of a close affinity with psychotherapy* has come true for our field. Two parallel forces appear in communication disorders—a strong humanistic force and an equally strong behavioral trend—which are reflected by the split in the journals between research and clinical articles as well as by the split in audiology between the rehabilitative audiologist and the diagnostic audiologist. Relatively few people are comfortable in both areas. Historically the field of communication disorders grew from humanistic roots. During the 1960s and the mid-1970s our field seemed to be dominated by a strong behavioral orientation. Recently there has been increasing evidence "that counseling procedures could be integrated with behavioral modification techniques" (Cooper, 1983) and perhaps the trend of the eighties will be an integration of these seemingly incompatible approaches.

---

*The term *psychotherapy* is used very loosely in the communication disorders literature, frequently synonymously with *counseling*. In this text, psychotherapy will denote a therapeutic relationship between a patient who has a chronic life-adjustment problem and a therapist who is usually a psychiatrist. At best, in practice the distinction between counseling and psychotherapy is a fuzzy one.

BEHAVIORAL AND HUMANISTIC
COUNSELING

The speech therapist/audiologist is confronted with an apparent choice in the selection of a model for changing behavior. On the one hand, there is the behavioral model that originated in the United States from the work of John Watson, with roots going back to Pavlov and his classically conditioned responses of the dog. Behaviorists concentrated on the strictly observable with emphasis on the external, environmental influences. This emphasis was in sharp contrast to the subjectivity of the Freudian movement, which was then beginning to invade American psychology. Strict behaviorists believe that humans are reactive beings whose behavior is controlled by external events: behavior is the product of a succession of reinforcements provided by others. Currently the leading proponent of behaviorism in the United States in B. F. Skinner, who is best known for his work with operant conditioning. Skinner contends that human behavior is shaped by the environment that "operates" on it; that is, if a particular behavior is rewarded—reinforced—by the environment, then that particular behavior will be repeated. Skinner has developed a widely used model of conditioning subjects using operant techniques.

A word about reinforcement, which is critical to the behaviorist notions: reinforcement is either positive as in giving a reward when the desired behavior is elicited, or negative as when an aversive stimulus is removed as a consequence of the individual's behavior. Negative reinforcement is not to be confused with punishment in which an aversive stimulus is applied as a consequence of behavior. The reinforcement, whether positive or negative, must be applied according to a schedule of reinforcement. The timing of the reinforcer must be precise, and the reinforcer must be either desirable to the individual or aversive enough to cause the behavior to change. The fact that the behavior of humans can be changed as a result of the systematic application of reinforcement can be demonstrated repeatedly, both in laboratory conditions and in actual living conditions.

The story is told, perhaps apocryphal, of a psychology professor who was lecturing her class on operant conditioning techniques when, unbeknown to her, the class decided to condition *her*. Every time she moved to the left, the class would sit up and take notes and appear to listen attentively; as soon as she moved to the right, they would slump in their seats. It was not long before she was lecturing from the doorway situated at the far left of the room. When the class got bored with this, they modified her behavior by reinforcing any movement to the right and she was soon to be found lecturing from the window. The professor, sophisticated though she was, responded much like a pigeon in a Skinner box, the apparent victim of the reinforcement schedule maintained by the class.

Parallel with the development of behaviorism in the United States (mid-twentieth century) was the development of humanistic psychology known as the "third force" in American psychology (third after Freudian psychoanalysis and Watsonian behaviorism). The theoretical and clinical underpinnings of the humanistic movement were provided by Rollo May, Carl Rogers, and Abraham Maslow. Maslow postulated that humans have an innate drive to grow and that this drive for what he termed *self-actualization* frequently is thwarted by inadequate teaching and parenting. The goal of therapy is to help the person remove the barriers and find that self-actualizing drive by responding to her own inner prompting where true wisdom lies. The means for releasing the self-actualizing drive can be through the relationship with the teacher/therapist. The notion that change is effected through relationship is essential to the humanistic point of view. Maslow's major breakthrough was in the application of this theory to normal people, since clinical psychiatry at that time was very much involved with identified patients who were emotionally ill.

Rogers, in particular, has done the most to demystify the counseling experience and to bring the fruits of clinical psychiatry to bear on the problems of the "normal" individual. His seminal work *Client Centered Therapy* (1951) marked an ideological turning point in the then contemporary clinical psychological movement, which at that time was highly committed to vocational counseling, mental testing, and personality evaluation. The client-centered counseling of Rogers placed little emphasis on diagnosis and testing, but stressed the quality of the interpersonal relationship. He also moved away from the doctor-patient model that prevailed in psychiatry and called the person to be counseled *client*. Rogers has continued writing and teaching extensively on what has become known as *person-centered therapy*.

In 1961, the American Association of Humanistic Psychology was founded; the Association president, James Bugental (1964), suggested five basic postulates.

1. Man, as man, supersedes the sum of his parts. (That is, man cannot be understood from a scientific study of part functions.)
2. Man has his being in a human context. (That is, man cannot be understood in part functions, which ignore interpersonal experiences.)
3. Man is aware (and cannot be understood by a psychology that fails to recognize man's continuous, many layered self-awareness).

4. Man has choice. (Man is not a bystander to his existence; he creates his own experience.)

5. Man is intentional. (Man points to the future: he has purpose, value, and meaning.)

Arbuckle (1970) later delineated the humanistic credo in counseling.

Man basically is free and any man can come to learn and to grow and to become the free person he is. This is the purpose of counseling, to help the individual to lose himself from his deterministic shackles and come to realize and to see what he has always had, choice and freedom (p. 35).

The reader can plainly see that a strict behaviorist would dispute almost all of the contentions of the humanists. For the behavioral psychologist, there is no freedom and choice. Change is due to external stimuli (i.e., which particular behavior is reinforced); the therapist must always stay with observable behavior; and a person does not act upon the world, the world acts upon the person. For the humanistic counselor, change is a function of growth (Maslow's inner drive for self-actualization as the motivation for change); the relationship is the basis for change; and undergirding all humanistic therapies is the notion that we are responsible for our own behavior.

To sharply contrast these points of view, a behaviorist might define a person as a collection of behaviors that have been reinforced by the environment, whereas a humanist defines the person as an organism seeking to grow. (Freudians might see a person as a series of repressed and sublimated instinctual drives.) These opposing philosophies tended to split the field of counseling during the 1960s and 1970s much as they had in communication disorders.

BEHAVIORISM AND HUMANISM
IN COMMUNICATION
DISORDERS

To the speech-language pathologist and audiologist, behavior modification can be a very attractive way of dealing with deviant behavior. It provides a structured framework by which the therapist can specify the particular behavior to be changed. By breaking down the task into a series of successive approximations and judiciously applying reinforcements, the deviant behavior can be modified. Progress at all stages can be readily measured. Perkins (1977) has commented:

> Because Speech Therapy is just as behavioral as behavior modification (the former derived pragmatically, the latter from operant learning principles) the same general therapeutic considerations underlie most of the methods for remediating speech. . . . In a word, the clinician must begin where his client can perform without failure and by careful selection of types and schedules of reinforcement, move step by step to the terminal goal. No step is taken until its success is assured. At the first sign of failure the therapist mounts a strategic retreat to a point at which successful performance can be established (p. 379).

It should be noted, however, that this approach presupposes a very narrow view of the speech therapist's role and responsibility, limiting the clinician to altering some very specific motor behavior. A highly mechanistic view of the speech-language pathologist's task, it also leaves unanswered the question of carryover into the client's environment where presumably a number of "reinforcers" are helping to maintain the deviant behavior.

Behavior modification techniques appear to be used quite extensively in communication disorders. For example, Shames and Florance (1982) recommend a behavioral approach to shaping fluency in young stutterers, while Moore (1982) recommends behavioral modification to eliminate or reduce vocal abuse. Cottrel

and colleagues (1980) utilize operant techniques for teaching vocabulary to developmentally delayed children. Operant techniques have been used extensively in audiology to condition difficult-to-test populations to respond to sound (Yarnell, 1982;
Lloyd, Spradlin, and Reid, 1968). The communication disorders
literature of the late sixties and seventies is rife with articles on
behavioral clinical approaches. There would be no advantage to
cite these studies at this point; however, two studies, I think, indicate the extent to which behavioral notions seemed to domi-
nate clinical speech pathology and audiology. These are the study
by Stech and colleagues (1973), which described the ways in
which the client reinforces and shapes the clinician's behavior
and—perhaps the ultimate in behaviorism in our field—Starkweather's (1974) scheme to reinforce the student clinician at the
precise moment that she is correctly reinforcing the client. (One
wonders who is reinforcing the supervisor.)

Speech pathology and audiology also have a long humanistic history going back to some of our earliest practitioners, which
seems to have been forgotten during the past decade. Van Riper
(1981) reports that Smiley Blanton, who opened the first speech
clinic in 1914, had a deep interest in psychotherapy but "never
became an orthodox Freudian." Backus and Beasley writing in
1951 felt that "Speech therapy more and more is shifting away
from an orientation based primarily upon devices, toward one
based primarily upon therapeutic relationships." Cooper (1966)
in his research on stutterers reports that client progress was related to the nature of the affect interchange between the client
and the clinician, and that important similarities exist between
stuttering therapy and psychotherapy. Webster (1966, 1977) has
consistently argued for a humanistic counseling model for the
speech pathologist/audiologist in relationship to parents. Caracciolo and colleagues (1978) attempted to use a Rogerian nondi-

rective approach in the supervision of student clinicans. Their hope was, by role-modeling the Rogerian helping relationship to the student clinician, that the would-be clinician could transfer this to the client relationship. Currently in the field of communication disorders, probably no one has been as consistently humanistic in both his clinical behavior and his writing as Albert Murphy (1982).

Happiness in this noblest sense comes in large measure through helping relationships with others, stretching our professional resources and the resources of the mind and heart. Every now and then something in our deeper selves enables us to realize that what truly counts in life is not a matter of what is in you or what is in me but of what occurs between us. That divine spark of relationship may be the most fundamental lifeforce of all (p. 473).

The problem with the humanistic approach is how to apply it to the field of communication disorders. The concepts are unclear and not readily amenable to scientific measurement; humanism requires a leap of faith that given the right conditions the self-actualizing drive will bubble through. Clinicians are left in an uncomfortable unstructured framework. They must learn behavior that appears to be contrary to what is usually thought of as being professional (i.e., listening as opposed to acting and prescribing). Gregory (1983) has commented in terms of counseling stutterers that:

It may be giving information expresses dominance and giving direction is related to manipulation and control. Whereas we may view listening and attempting to understand as being indecisive and uncertain. For whatever reason, many student clinicians and professional speech language pathologists seem to find it easier to be a provider of information and direction (p. 10).

A humanistic approach is very demanding of the therapist and there is no clinical evidence to indicate that it will modify speech behavior any better than behavioral techniques. How then is the clinician to resolve this apparent split between the behaviorist and humanist? I think the split in practice is becoming more theoretical than real, although there are some very real differences. In much of current behavioral counseling (post-Skinner), the therapists have come to recognize that one of the first goals of the counselor is to establish a relationship with the client such that the client feels free to express herself to the counselor, and in which the client perceives the counselor as someone who is interested in attempting to help her with her problems. The relationship between the counselor and the client needs to be nonjudgmental so that the client will feel free to discuss her problems. It is also the client who selects the goals of therapy and, in concert with the therapist, works to change the environmental reinforcers that are maintaining the current self-defeating behavior (Hansen, Stavis, and Warner, 1977). This view of counseling becomes more acceptable to the humanistic stance; in fact, at times, it seems very person-centered. Rogers (1961), for example, has stated that it is not the theoretical or technical orientation of the therapist but rather the attitudes and feelings that determine the quality of the personal interaction that determines growth. Presumably Rogers could accept a "behavioral" counselor who established a nonjudgmental relationship with her client and who listened empathically. It is also impossible to know just what single element or elements in the relationship are responsible for promoting change.

The humanist cannot deny the role of conditioning in determining human behavior. Yalom (1975) (no behaviorist, he) has commented that "every form of psychotherapy is a learning process relying in part on operant conditioning." By this he seems to mean the social reinforcers that are used almost unconsciously by the therapist/teacher. So much of our early learning is based on social approval and on the nonsystematic application of operant techniques that most adults become approval-seeking. Therapists use this approval-seeking as a means of reinforcing the desired behavior. The humanistic counselor, however, does not systematically and consciously set out to control the other in a relationship. Nonetheless there are controlling elements in all humanistic encounters, some of which are based on operant procedures.

Clearly, we do have choices and we can resist environmental reinforcers. If the college professor alluded to earlier had become aware of what the class was trying to do to her, she could have resisted their conditioning and lectured from the center of the room, albeit discomfited by the fact that she was talking to a group of students who appeared to be asleep. She could also have elected to talk to them about what was happening and negotiated the differences between them. I think it is clear that we are, in part, controlled by our environment and in part, control it. It is our awareness of what is happening to us and our willingness to assume responsibility for how we behave that will enable us to control environmental reinforcers.

We cannot entirely avoid the operant paradigm (nor should we) in communication disorders. Much to my humanistic chagrin, I find that I use operant techniques and constructs frequently. For example, in the nursery, when we have separated a child from her mother and the child begins to cry, we do not allow the mother (who is watching from a one-way mirror) to go directly into the nursery because this would "reinforce" the crying behavior. Instead, we wait until the child is happy, or at least quiet, and then allow the mother to enter. (Of course, a true humanist would not separate the mother and child until both are ready to make the break; however, this might take considerable time and programatic exigencies dictate a quick separation. Such are the compromises that a clinician must make.)

There are however, some real differences between behavioral thinking and humanistic thinking as well as differences in attitudes toward personal responsibility. Robert Pirsig, in his perhaps classic book *Zen and the Art of Motorcycle Maintenance*, distinguished between a romantic and a classical thinker. The classical thinker would see a motorcycle and would be interested in how the parts went together to make it move; the romantic looking at the same motorcycle would see transportation. Romantic thinking is inspirational, imaginative, and intuitive; classical thinking is straightforward, unemotional, economical, and unadorned. One can safely substitute right-brain left-brain thinking or, I think, humanistic versus behavioral thinking. Humanists tend to be of the romantic variety and behaviorists of the classical. One way of thinking is not necessarily better than the other, they are just different ways of looking at the same thing. The trick is to integrate both and to be comfortable in both modes of thinking—a difficult feat to achieve. As a field, we must provide room for both kinds of thinking and come to value the contributions that each mode of thinking can bring to the profession.

The second area where behaviorists and humanists differ is in responsibility assumption. In all behavioral therapies the relationship bewteen client and counselor is not equal. The therapist is perceived as having more information and wisdom than the client. At some point the counselor assumes responsibility for controlling or helping to control (albeit at the client's behest) the client's behavior. In addition, the counselor generally accepts the major responsibility for deciding on the particular course of therapy and accepts the responsibility for its outcome (Hansen, Stavis, and Warner, 1977).

On the other hand, the humanistic orientation assumes an equality in the relationship with the client having equal power. The clinician trusts the client to make responsible decisions and to assume responsibility for the course of therapy. Wisdom lies within the individual and the therapist's role is to help the person find and tune into her own wisdom. The clinician's responsibility is limited to creating the proper environment for growth to take place.

Central to the distinction between behavioral and humanistic counseling is the notion of locus of control. Rotter (1966) developed a scale that measures whether an individual has an internal or external locus of control. People with an internal locus of control tend to feel that they have power and can control their personal destiny. Externals, on the other hand, feel that they are controlled by others. Within the sphere of humanistic counseling, control is always vested within the client and not the therapist. Behaviorists tend to feel that control is external to the individual and that it is a matter of finding the right reinforcers in order to achieve the desired behavioral objective.

Belief in an inner locus of control is not a dichotomous variable but rather one that is on a continuum. There is, however, some point where one believes in and encourages in others an inner (as opposed to an external) locus of control. It is at that point that one may move from a behavioral set to a humanistic point of view. The notion of locus of control is central to all counseling and will be discussed in greater detail in subsequent chapters.

This book is written from what I hope can be seen as a thoroughgoing humanistic point of view with a nod of respect to the formidable contributions of the behaviorists. The humanistic point of view fits my temperament (I was not a machine person). For me the joy—the noble happiness that Murphy speaks about—is within the caring relationship provided by the humanist frame of reference; it is also a "burnout" preventer. I also think that the subjective concept of self-actualization holds more promise for the therapeutic growth of both clinician and client, and ultimately for our field, than does the rather mechanistic and deterministic view of the behaviorists. It is the willingness of the therapist to both transcend a strict behaviorism and integrate behavioral notions with humanism that distinguishes the clinician from the technician. Each of us in our clinical interaction must make a choice as to how we want to view the clinician-client relationship—a choice that needs to be made with both thought and awareness.

Rogers (1980), quoting the 2,500-year-old words of Chinese sage Lao-Tse, captures the essence of the humanistic point of view in relationships:

> If I keep from meddling with people, they take care of themselves.
> If I keep from commanding people, they behave themselves.
> If I keep from preaching at people, they improve themselves.
> If I keep from imposing on people, they become themselves.

BIBLIOGRAPHY

Arbuckle, D. S. *Counseling: Philosophy, Theory and Practice* (2nd ed.). Boston: Allyn & Bacon, 1970.

Backus, O., and Beasley, J. *Speech Therapy with Children*. Cambridge, Mass.: Houghton Mifflin, 1951.

Blanchard, S. Current practices in the counseling of the laryngectomy patient. *J. Commun. Disord.* 15:233, 1982.

Bugental, J. F. T. The third force in psychology. *J. Humanistic Psychol.* 1:4, 1964.

Caracciolo, G., Rigrodsky, S., and Morrison, E. A Rogerian orientation to the speech-language pathology supervision relationship. *ASHA* 20:286, 1978.

Clark, J. Counseling in a pediatric audiologic practice. *ASHA* 24:521, 1982.

Cooper, E. Client-clinician relationships and concomitant factors in stuttering therapy. *J. Speech Hear. Disord.* 9:194, 1966.

Cooper, E. *Understanding the Process in Counseling Stutterers.* Memphis: Speech Foundation of America, publication no. 18, 1983.

Cottrel, A., Montague, J., Farb, J., and Throne, S. An operant procedure for improving vocabulary definition performance in developmentally delayed children. *J. Speech Hear. Disord.* 45:90, 1980.

Gregory, H. *The Clinician's Attitudes in Counseling Stutterers.* Memphis: Speech Foundation of America, publication no. 18, 1983.

Hansen, J., Stavis, R., and Warner, R. *Counseling Theory and Process.* Boston: Allyn & Bacon, 1977.

Lloyd, L., Spradlin, J., and Reid, M. An operant audiometric procedure for difficult-to-test patients. *J. Speech Hear. Disord.* 33:236, 1968.

Moore, P. Voice Disorders. In G. Shames and E. Wig (Eds.), *Human Communication Disorders.* Columbus, Ohio: Merrill, 1982.

Murphy, A. The Clinical Process and the Speech-Language Pathologist. In G. Shames and E. Wig (Eds.), *Human Communication Disorders.* Columbus, Ohio: Merrill, 1982.

Panbacker, M. Parental preoperative ideas of speech after surgical management of cleft palate. *Rehabil. Lit.* 38:352, 1977.

Perkins, W. P. *Speech Pathology: An Applied Behavioral Science* (2nd ed.). St. Louis: Mosby, 1977.

Pirsig, R. *Zen and the Art of Motorcycle Maintenance.* New York: Morrow, 1974.

Rogers, C. *Client Centered Therapy.* Boston: Houghton Mifflin 1951.

Rogers, C. *On Becoming a Person.* Boston: Houghton Mifflin, 1961.

Rogers, C. *A Way of Being.* Boston: Houghton Mifflin, 1980.

Rotter, J. Generalized expectancies for internal versus external control of reinforcement. *Psychol. Monogr. General and Applied,* 80, No. 1, Whole No. 609, 1966.

Shames, G., and Florance, C. Disorders of Fluency. In G. Shames and E. Wig. (Eds.), *Human Communication Disorders.* Columbus, Ohio: Merrill, 1982.

Starkweather, C. Behavior modification in training speech clinicians: Procedures and implications. *ASHA* 16:607, 1974.

Stech, E., Curtiss, J., Troesch, P., and Binnie, C. Clients' reinforcement of speech clinicians: A factor-analytic study. *ASHA* 15:287, 1973.

Tanner, D. C. Loss and grief: Implication for the speech-language pathologist and audiologist. *ASHA* 22:916, 1980.

Travis, L. E. The Psychotherapeutic Process. In L. E. Travis (Ed.), *Handbook of Speech Pathology.* New York: Appleton-Century-Crofts, 1957.

Van Riper, C. An early history of ASHA. *ASHA* 23:855, 1981.

Webster, E. Parent counseling by speech pathologists and audiologists. *J. Speech Hear. Disord.* 31:331, 1966.

Webster, E. *Counseling with Parents of Handicapped Children.* New York: Grune & Stratton, 1977.

Yalom, I. D. *The Theory and Practice of Group Psychotherapy* (2nd ed.). New York: Basic Books, 1975.

Yarnell, G. Comparison of operant and conventional audiometric procedures with multihandicapped (deaf-blind) children. *Volta Rev.* 85:69, 1983.

CHAPTER 2

EXISTENTIAL ISSUES
IN COUNSELING THE
COMMUNICATIVELY
DISORDERED

Paralleling the development of humanism in the United States was the growth of existential philosophy in Europe. The "existentialists" emerged on the rediscovery by the French intellectual movement of the work of the mid-nineteenth century philosopher Kierkegaard. Philosopher/poets such as Sartre and Camus articulated and in effect popularized the existential philosophy in plays and novels. They were attempting to look at the problems of human existence without the comfort provided by traditional religious thought. To the existentialist the problems of living are related to facts of existence, namely that we must die, that we have choices, that we are alone, and that life is meaningless. These notions are painful and most people want to retreat from examining life as viewed by the existentialists.

The existential ideas also became the basis of an approach to psychotherapy. Therapists such as Frankl, Fromm, and May began to use the existential philosophy as a basis for understanding and examining the problems presented to them by their patients. Almost all of the existential therapists were latter-day psychoanalysts. In traditional psychoanalytic thought, anxiety is seen as the motivating force. The source of anxiety is the conflict that is generated between instinctual drives, such as thanatos (death) and eros (life), or between the id (pleasure drive) and the social restrictions as incorporated within the infant in the form of the conscience (superego). The resultant anxiety from these conflicts is the source of neurotic behavior. Existential psychotherapy is also a dynamic therapy that postulates anxiety as the motivating force. For the existential psychotherapists, however, the anxiety occurs when the individual confronts the givens of existence, namely death, responsibility, loneliness, and meaninglessness. In order to cope with this anxiety the individual develops defense mechanisms that lead to neurotic behavior. The task of the therapist is to help the person come to grips with the givens of existence in a healthy and constructive manner. First, however, the therapist must learn to deal with his own anxiety. Existential therapists do not take a developmental view of behavior; that is, they are not especially concerned with promoting insight into the person's early history in order to understand the client's current behavior. Instead they focus on the present and on how the patient is dealing with the facts of existence.

There does not appear to be any one set of therapeutic techniques that distinguishes this school from others. To some extent all psychotherapists are existentialists in that they must focus at some point on what "is." The existentialists differ from the humanists because they tend to stress the limitations of existence and to be more philosophically pessimistic. Humanists, on the other hand, are generally very upbeat, positive, and affirming. In the main, humanistic psychologists are comfortable within an existential framework; the two schools are very closely allied, especially around the issue of responsibility assumption.

In an absolute gem of a book, *Existential Psychotherapy*, Irvin Yalom has merged the existential philosophy and contemporary American psychotherapy. There is not yet any formal organization of existential therapists as occurred with the humanistic psychologists in the 1960s. Presently they appear to be a loose collection of psychotherapists who think along similar lines. The movement needs a unifying document, and Yalom's book may provide such an impetus. I suspect that the fourth force emerging in the 1980s in American psychotherapy will be the existential movement.

The existential notions of death, responsibility, loneliness, and meaninglessness also appear to have cogency for the field of communication disorders. Practicing speech pathologists deal with death in many different forms such as providing therapy for individuals who have had a recent encounter with the death experience (e.g., stroke victims), or counseling the parents of a disabled child who mourn the loss of the dream of having a normal child. All therapeutic relationships must deal with the termination issue. Responsibility assumption is a vital consideration for any therapeutic change. Loneliness is a given experience of anyone with a communication disorder. The resolution of the meaninglessness issue provides the life direction for the individual; people who undergo catastrophic change must find for themselves some meaning in the event and a new direction for their lives.

This chapter will first deal briefly with each existential issue—death, responsibility, loneliness, and meaninglessness—as viewed by the philosophers, showing its possible application to the field of communication disorders.

D E A T H

Probably the single most important event of life is death; yet this is a topic that most people avoid. The surest way I know to create an uncomfortable audience is to bring up the topic of death. Our society seems to be predicated on death avoidance. I think that the cartoon of a husband talking to his wife with the caption "If one of us should die before the other, I think I will move to Paris," demonstrates the underlying anxiety about death, which is perhaps universal. In *The American Way of Death*, Jessica Mitford points out how funeral directors cater to our death avoidance—and thereby increase their profits on funerals—by providing elegant clothing for the deceased, a soft and buoyant mattress, and, of course, the marvelous euphemism of a "slumber room" for the last viewing of the elegant coffin that contains the "sleeping" corpse.

The existential philosophers, on the other hand, tell us that with death awareness comes a more total awareness and appreciation of life. Encountering death is a "boundary experience," a time when a person can look at everyday existence and can shift from the everyday reality in which he may sleepwalk through the day to a more intense reality. Boundary experiences are those events that push us into a more intense awareness of our existence. Persons who live with death awareness savor and enjoy every moment of the day. They are aware of how transitory and finite life is; they do not squander their time.

Carlos Castaneda has written a series of books published within the last 15 years that have an almost cult status. Castaneda was an anthropology student who attempted to study the Mexican

Indian culture with an eye to discovering how they used hallucinogenic drugs in their religious rituals. He inadvertently became apprenticed to a sorcerer, don Juan, who, at least in the first books of the series, used an astonishing variety of teaching techniques. The books contain many dialogues between Carlos and don Juan in which the sorcerer expands quite clearly on European existential philosophy. No nondirective counselor is he; here he is on death, which is one of his favorite topics.

"Death is the only wise adviser that we have. Whenever you feel as you always do, that everything is going wrong and you're about to be annihilated, turn to your death and ask if that is so. Your death will tell you that you're wrong; that nothing really matters outside its touch. Your death will tell you, 'I haven't touched you yet.' " . . .

"It is meaningless. If it [death] is out there waiting for me, why should I worry about it?"

"I didn't say you had to worry about it."

"What am I supposed to do then?"

"Use it. Focus your attention on the link between you and your death, without remorse or sadness or worrying. Focus your attention on the fact that you don't have time and let your act flow accordingly. Only under these conditions will your acts have their rightful power. Otherwise they will be for as long as you live, the acts of a timid man. . . . Our death is waiting and this very act we're performing now may very well be our last battle (I call it a battle on earth because it is a struggle). Most people move from act to act without any struggle or thought" (1972, p. 111).

It is the idea of death that makes it possible for us to live life in an authentic fashion. Without the notion of death, life loses its intensity; we mark time as we kill an hour or we are bored. When we live with death awareness, we know that each moment is precious and is not to be wasted. Life is replete with terminations: these are symbolic deaths. For example, I became a much better parent the day that my oldest child left home. Her departure brought home to me in a very forceful way how fleeting our relationships are. Active parenting—like life—is a transitory experience, to be enjoyed and savored and then we move on.

Yalom (1980) found the following changes in the lives of cancer patients, as they come to grips with their impending death:

A rearrangement of life's priorities; a trivializing of the trivial

A sense of liberation; being able to choose not to do those things that they do not wish to do

An enhanced sense of living in the immediate present rather than postponing life until retirement or some other part of the future

A vivid appreciation of the elemental facts of life; the changing seasons, the wind, falling leaves, the last Christmas, and so forth

Deeper communication with loved ones than before the crisis

Fewer interpersonal fears, less concern about rejection, greater willingness to take risks than before the crisis

Would that we could all develop death awareness without having cancer. Unfortunately death awareness for many people seems to come about only as a result of a particular crisis.

The professional in the field of communication disorders very frequently is working with people who are in the midst of such a life crisis. The stroke victim and laryngectomized person come immediately to mind. Webster (1982), a speech pathologist who suffered a cerebrovascular accident (stroke), found that with recovery things like "trees, flowers, sunsets, and friends and loved ones—are more appreciated." However, anyone who sustains a grievous loss such as parents of disabled children, who must give up the dream of having a normal child, will also undergo something very similar to the death experience. They are also very much in crisis, and it is how the professional deals with this crisis that can facilitate growth and the shifting of life priorities that accompanies these crises.

Tanner (1980) has written a comprehensive article on the grief reaction and how this relates to the speech pathologist/audiologist. He comments that loss can be both real and symbolic, and that grief is not a single reaction but is a complex progression involving many emotions and attempts to cope with loss.

One cannot talk about death and grieving without mentioning the work of Kübler-Ross (1969). She has described extensively five stages of the grief process: (1) denial, (2) anger, (3) bargaining, (4) depression, and (5) acceptance. Although this model is useful for understanding the process that parents of disabled children go through, one has to be careful about oversimplifying a very complex process. I have used this model in my writings and lectures and find it useful for understanding the general behavior of grief. A given parent, however, handles the grief reaction in unique ways that clinicians must be prepared to meet. Helen Featherstone, the parent of a severely disabled child and the author of *A Difference in the Family*, has caught this problem quite well.

But I am uncomfortable with most stage theories, they carry too heavy a freight of straight line progress; they also suggest an implausible final harmony. The actual progress is not linear, and often is bought at a high price in human suffering. In the vocabulary of stages, acceptance becomes a kind of high plateau, once out of reach, now firmly felt underfoot. Gone are the fears and self-reproaches of yesterday and sighs for what might have been. Matter of fact realism guides our effort. Having struggled out of darkness, we will not have to be afraid anymore. . . .

Few parents reach an emotional promised land; most have good days and bad days (1980, p. 232).

Acceptance does not signify an end to pain—one cannot suffer a grievous loss without travail. Even when acceptance is won, there are still bad times. What does seem to happen to parents and to those undergoing a severe crisis is that they eliminate the pettiness of life. A shifting of values occurs as when one encounters death; parents come to recognize what is truly important and that they do not have time to worry about trivialities.

Death awareness mobilizes the individual. When you are aware that death can touch you at any time, you abandon timidity. You wish to extract the most from every encounter and you recognize that nothing is permanent. For the clinician, termination becomes an important clinical tool. All meetings need to have a very definite closure. It is no accident that parent groups become more intense as the hour for termination draws near or when the participants become aware of the term ending. Relationships become more intense at termination; one only has to stand in an airport and watch people say goodbye to realize the intensity of feeling surrounding termination awareness. Clients will be motivated to work hard when they know that they have a very limited time to be with the clinician. There is experimental support for these notions: Shlien and colleagues (1962) found that patients within a time-limited counseling program made more progress than did patients within a counseling program that had no time limits imposed. This was true of both Adlerian and client-centered therapy. Munro and Bach (1975) found that college students seeking counseling services showed significantly more gains in self-acceptance and increased independence in time-limited therapy (eight sessions) than did a control group of students who had no time limitation placed on them.

When both clinician and client recognize that there is limited time, the emphasis in therapy becomes quality of endeavor. Time per se does not heal, only activity does. With an awareness of time limitation comes an increase in activity and risk; therefore, time limitation can be a very vital clinical tool.

Through death awareness we can restore our zest in our work, for clinicians who live with death awareness cannot be bored. They recognize that there is only limited time and they extract the most from each therapy session and the most from the relationships that they establish.

Each of the other existential issues contributes to further understanding of the therapeutic process. Responsibility assumption will lead to change and growth; through loneliness we find love; and the resolution of meaninglessness gives rise to commitment.

RESPONSIBILITY

The existentialists are unyielding on the issue of responsibility. You are entirely responsible for your life and for constituting your reality. You are responsible for all your feelings—nobody makes you feel anything. You are also responsible for your dreams, desires, and, above all else, your own happiness (not only for your actions but for what you fail to do). This uncompromising position can leave you very uncomfortable because there is no one to blame but yourself. For example, you are responsible for the plight of the American Indians because you made a choice not to contribute to relief efforts, you chose not to mobilize others to raise funds, and you chose to ignore the problem. There is no moral judgment—never a statement that you should do anything about the Indians—just that you have not done anything about it, therefore, you are responsible.

As one might expect, don Juan has much to say about responsibility.

"Since the day you were born, one way or another, someone has been doing something to you," he said.

"That's correct," I said.

"And they have been doing something to you against your will."

"True."

"And by now you are helpless, like a leaf in the wind."

"That's correct, that's the way it is."

I said that the circumstances of my life had sometimes been devastating. He listened attentively but I could not figure out whether he was just being agreeable or genuinely concerned until I noticed that he was trying to hide a smile.

"No matter how much you like to feel sorry for yourself you have to change that," he said in a soft tone. "It doesn't jibe with the life of a warrior." . . .

"The hardest thing in the world is to assume the mood of a warrior," he said. "It is of no use to be sad and complain and feel justified in doing so, believing that someone is always doing something to us. Nobody is doing anything to anybody much less a warrior. You are here with me, because you want to be here. You should have assumed full responsibility by now, so that the idea that you are here at the mercy of the wind is inadmissible (1972, p. 139)."

One can no longer "blame the wind" or others for one's behavior. When I have to take full responsibility for myself and all my perceptions, then I may feel very anxious (also very alone). The discomfort in responsibility assumption is that it leaves me open to guilt, for if I am responsible, then I have only myself to blame if anything goes wrong. Guilt is such an uncomfortable feeling that it is easy to try to repress it or to displace the blame onto someone else. Guilt is generally defined as "anxiety plus a sense of badness." Guilty people are generally very difficult to work with as they tend to stew with their guilt and to not act. Guilt, because it is such an uncomfortable feeling, also breeds resentment. Relationships that are built around guilt seldom flourish.

There are three kinds of guilt: neurotic guilt, real guilt, and existential guilt. Neurotic guilt is the guilt we feel for events that we are not in any logical way responsible for; this generalized guilt feeling leaves individuals very unhappy and very uncomfortable. Some people seem to pick up guilt as a magnet picks up iron filings. This seems to be particularly true of the mothers of handicapped children. Guilt implies power; when I feel guilty (as opposed to being responsible in the existential sense) for the American Indian, my guilt implies that I can do something about it.

Neurotic guilt is very often the way that the powerless can feel power and can control others—as distorted as that may seem. By giving others the power to hurt them, they can control the other person in the relationship. Thus the parent who tells the child how much the child's behavior hurts him can be developing neurotic guilt in the child. Although this action seems to give the child a great deal of power, in actuality it limits the child through his guilt feelings and desire to not hurt the parent. Guilt is a very complex issue. When self-esteem is enhanced and people begin to feel their own power (inner locus of control) then neurotic guilt is given up.

Real guilt occurs when we have committed an actual transgression against another and, in order to feel better, we make restitution where possible. In the film *Gandhi* a Hindu man approaches the fasting Gandhi and tells him that he has killed a

Moslem child. Gandhi's response was "I have a solution for you. You must adopt a Moslem child who has no parents and you must raise it as a Moslem." The notion of expiation of sins through restitution is an ancient one and the Catholic church confessional and the Yom Kippur week of atonement of the Jews are both means designed to relieve real guilt through expiation. Probably the cruelest thing that we can do in a relationship is not to allow someone who has wronged us in some way to pay us back. When we do that we are telling him to stew in his own guilt.

For the existential therapist, however, there is a third kind of guilt: the guilt we feel when we transgress against ourselves or when we fail to respond to our self-actualizing drive, known as existential guilt. This is another point at which humanism and existentialism overlap. An individual who fails to live as fully as he can, and fails to develop potential, will experience existential guilt. The trick with existential guilt is to respond to it. It is a call from ourselves to ourselves to grow. The discomfort caused by the existential guilt can be a vital spur to increasing our willingness to take risks and to change.

Responsibility assumption also has a very positive side in that we can also take credit for all the good things we do. During the course of a lifetime the vast majority of decisions made by most people are good ones. Yet in my clinical experience people are generally reluctant to take the credit for the good decisions and are only too eager to take the blame for the bad. These are the people who attribute the good in their life to "luck"; all the bad was their responsibility. This view can lead to a rather unhappy life and seems to be a concomitant of low self-esteem individuals.

I do not think that it is necessary to accept the extreme position of the existentialist: that we are responsible for everything that happens to us. I, for example, cannot see how one is responsible for having a congenital birth defect. We do, however, have to take responsibility for how we respond to what happens to us. We can choose to grow from adversity and make it a positive event, or we can feel sorry for ourselves. We have a choice as to how we wish to see things—our glass can be either half full or half empty. David Wright, a poet and a deafened adult, has written elegantly about his deafness and about the handicapped. He can find many positives.

The handicapped are less at the mercy of vague unhappiness that afflicts so many, especially those without aim in life, whose consequent boredom promotes what used to be called spleen. The disabled have been given a built-in, ready-packed objective which is always present; a definite impediment to get the better of. Like the prospect of hanging it concentrates the faculties wonderfully (1969, p. 111).

Another example is Terry Fox, an 18-year-old boy who had his leg amputated because of cancer. At that point he could have chosen to be a cripple. Instead he set off on a trans-Canada run to raise money for the Canadian Cancer Society and, in the process, galvanized a whole country. The cancer killed Fox before he completed his run, but he did raise more than 10 million dollars and inspired many with his courage. We may not have much to say about which cards are dealt to us in life; however, we do have much to say about how we play those cards.

The pathology of responsibility evasion can range from the profound to the commonplace, and in some way, more or less, we all evade or try to evade responsibility. Erich Fromm (1941), in his classic book *Escape from Freedom*, has pointed out on a societal level that freedom engenders anxiety; hence, the rise of totalitarian forms of government as a protection against the responsibility required to maintain a democracy. There is probably no more common occurrence of responsibility evasion than in the addicted personality, the smoker or the alcoholic. Smoking or drinking is not something that happens to a person; it is something a person does to himself, yet smokers and drinkers seldom see that simple truth. For the past several years I have been working with groups of people who are trying to stop smoking. It is very clear to me that the smoker takes little if any responsibility for his own behavior. "I have to have a cigarette"; "No, you choose to have a cigarette," becomes a familiar litany within the group. No change will occur unless there is responsibility assumption, because the smoker is waiting for something from outside himself to happen. He is waiting for the "ultimate rescuer."

The idea of the ultimate rescuer is a juvenile belief system rooted in childhood. As young children we are saved repeatedly by the timely intervention of our parents. This belief system is carried over into our fantasy life and is best exemplified by films with happy endings, such as the "Perils of Pauline," where the heroine is always rescued at the last minute, or by Prince Charming in all his manifestations. Although these fantasies are very satisfying and persistent, it is our willingness to give them up that determines our maturity. For the adult there is no ultimate rescuer; there is the recognition that we are alone and we are responsible for our behavior. This realization can be very frightening psychologically because, ultimately, we have no one to count on but ourselves.

Smokers who are going to succeed in quitting seem quickly to assume responsibility for their own behavior, recognizing that nobody is going to make the change for them. Then they recognize that they are choosing to smoke. If they wish, they can make another choice for themselves. (They must also come to see that "not smoking" is not a deprivation but is rather a gift they give themselves.) Once they have these two notions, the cessation of smoking becomes relatively easy. In the same way I think that it is not helpful to think of alcoholism as a disease. There is no disease that I know of that requires someone to purchase a bottle and drink its contents—that is volition. While an alcoholic might metabolize alcohol differently than other people, he must still take responsibility for the drinking behavior itself if any change is to occur.

The humanistic and existentialist psychologists agree fully on the issue of responsibility assumption, and it is the essence of counseling. In a sense, all therapists agree on responsibility assumption because there can be no therapeutic change without it. The therapeutic question becomes how best to get the client to assume responsibility.

Another way of talking about responsibility assumption is locus of control. Persons with an inner locus of control will readily assume responsibility for their own behavior while those with a more external locus of control will attribute their behavior to forces outside themselves (i.e., fate, luck, or some higher power); seldom do they see their behavior as a choice they have made.

The communication disorders literature is fairly sparse concerning locus of control even though this is a vital therapeutic issue. Shirlberg and colleagues (1977) looked at locus of control in communication disorders majors and found that students who have an internal locus of control were rated as the better clinicians. As they so aptly put it, "Excellent clinicians do, in fact, view themselves as pilots rather than pawns of their fate." White

(1982) reports on a series of workshops he conducted with teachers and counselors at six schools for the deaf. Two-hundred-eighty-one participants were asked to rank 24 social competencies among the deaf. Almost all participants ranked "accepting responsibility for own actions" as the single most important issue for deaf students. Bodner and Johns (1977) used the Rotter scale on 38 high-reading deaf students and their hearing controls. They found that the deaf students were significantly more external in their locus of control than the normally hearing subjects. Dowaliby and associates (1983), in a series of studies conducted at the National Institute for the Deaf, administered a constructed learning style inventory test to 267 entering students and to a control sample of 100 normally hearing undergraduates. The test was a paper and pencil test that measured internality, externality, and people-orientation. Results indicated that the hearing-impaired students are substantially more external in their locus of control than the normally hearing students.

The failure to take responsibility for one's actions in the adult deaf population was recently and vividly brought home to me. I lectured at a conference attended by a large number of deaf adults, and my speech was consequently interpreted. After the speech, which was an hour's duration, a deaf adult complained that he could not see the interpreter and therefore had missed the whole speech. The conference organizer, whom I spoke to afterwards, felt bad and guilty about the incident until we talked about it. She then realized that the responsibility was his. He could have moved his seat or complained at the outset and the interpreter could have moved. Instead he chose to sit there and then complain about it.

The deaf individuals' external locus of control is mirrored in other disabled populations. For example, Hallahan and colleagues (1978) found that 28 matched learning-disabled teenagers were significantly more external in their control orientation than the normal subjects, while Land and Vineberg (1965) reported that blind subjects were more externally oriented than their sighted control subjects.

The finding of an external locus of control in disabled populations is not surprising. One would predict that disabled persons would feel that others are more powerful than they are, and that the control of their lives is outside of themselves. They are often dependent on others for many things. They are, however, helped in this attitude by professionals and by their own families who "rescue" the disabled. Geri Jewell, an actress with cerebral palsy, hearing loss, and a speech defect, feels that the biggest impediment to her growing up was that teachers had low expectations for her and did not require her to assume responsibility (*ASHA* interview, 1983).

Probably the best example of the ultimate rescuer in contemporary literature is the Annie Sullivan story. *Helen and Teacher*, a comprehensive biography of the relationship between Annie and Helen Keller written by Joseph Lash. Annie Sullivan had a very deprived childhood. After her mother's death, the 6-year-old Annie was placed in the poorhouse by her father. Her 4-year-old brother died shortly after being placed in the facility, and Annie literally had nothing, growing up among destitute, elderly people. Because of a visual problem Annie was sent to the Perkins School for the Blind in Boston and received her education among a blind population. The plea for help from the Kellers arrived as Annie was graduating, and she was sent to Alabama to rescue the family. It is easy to imagine the young Annie Sullivan as a descending angel or, to use another children's storybook character, Mary Poppins. She certainly must have seemed this way to the desperate Kellers who had an out-of-control deaf and blind child.

And as Mary Poppins would have done, Annie quickly brought order to the house. She took Helen to a shack on the property, literally strapped Helen to her at night, and proceeded to civilize her. The movie and play *The Miracle Worker* written by Gibson, which is based essentially on the same material that was available to Lash, ends with Annie's triumphant return from the shack. All of the viewers know that Helen turned out to be a truly remarkable person who achieved a great deal despite her disability, and it is tempting to conclude that they lived happily ever after.

The Lash biography, however, continues the story. The effect on Mrs. Keller was profound. In a short time this young woman from Boston accomplished more than she could in the years she tried to manage Helen. In effect, Mrs. Keller abandoned any attempt to actively mother Helen after that and seemed to be reduced to the role of a loving aunt. Annie's success convinced Mrs. Keller that she was a very inadequate mother for such a disabled child.

Helen and Annie went back to Boston and achieved all the outward manifestations of success, including graduation from Radcliffe College. However, such a closely dependent relationship in which Annie had almost all the control could not work in Helen's best interest (nor in Annie's). Annie could not let her be independent; in many ways she needed Helen more than Helen needed her. Annie's marriage foundered, in part because Annie would not give up her "little darling." After Annie's death, Helen went through a succession of companions, none of whom were completely able to satisfy her. She never learned how to live independently despite her formidable and remarkable skills.

I think that the failure to develop independent living skills was a direct function of the rescuing by Annie. Annie did not or could not allow Helen to be independent of her. It was not a happy ending.

Hornyak (1980), using the language of transactional analysis, has pointed out the dangers for the speech pathologists in "rescuing" clients. Rescuing robs people of their autonomy and keeps them feeling powerless and controlled. In the therapy contract Hornyak cautions that the client should be "perceived as a human being who is not helpless." When professionals become the ultimate rescuers of the disabled population they are servicing, they limit growth and keep the others from assuming responsibility for their own behavior. The notion of developing an inner locus of control in the client population is fundamental to the therapeutic process. Somehow we must teach the stutterers to take responsibility for their nonfluency, the dysphonics for their vocal behavior, and the articulatory defectives for their misarticulations. They must come to realize that change occurs from the inside rather than from external sources. When clients recognize their own powers and responsibilities, the specific speech behaviors can be altered, and the changes can be maintained outside the therapeutic relationship.

L O N E L I N E S S

Each of us is alone in the universe—after birth we can no longer merge with anyone else. At best we can communicate through a rather cumbersome symbol system, which requires several energy transformations and is very open to failure at any number of levels. This existential loneliness is a major source of anxiety. Almost all anxiety stems from the awareness of separation; the infant cannot bear to be separated from his parents, because separation can lead to death, and so the terror of loneliness is born. All change is a loneliness experience as we give up the comfort of the familiar. Yet we are alone—no relationship can eliminate isolation—and that crushing fact is central to existential thought.

In addition to the existential loneliness, an interpersonal loneliness occurs when we are cut off from contact with others and an intrapersonal loneliness occurs when we cut off parts of ourselves from our own consciousness. Awareness and fear of our aloneness can give rise to anxiety loneliness.

Loneliness is very much tied to death and responsibility. When we reflect on our death we become aware that we will die alone, no one can die for us. When we assume full responsibility we also become acutely aware of our loneliness. Moustakes (1961) is a psychologist who has written extensively about the loneliness experience and how it relates to psychotherapy. His awareness of existential loneliness came via the responsibility route when he had to make a decision regarding major surgery for his young daughter.

It was a terrible responsibility, being required to make a decision, a life or death decision, for someone else. This awful feeling, this overwhelming sense of responsibility, I could not share with anyone. I felt utterly alone, entirely lost and frightened; my existence was absorbed in the crisis. No one fully understood my terror or how this terror gave impetus to deep feelings of loneliness and isolation which had been dormant within me. There at the center of my being, loneliness aroused me to a self awareness I had never known before (p. 2).

Another way of experiencing existential loneliness is through an intense experience with interpersonal loneliness. Moustakes describes individuals who had experienced extreme isolation and wrote about their reaction to the experience. The common thread running through the accounts of explorers, lost seamen, or downed pilots was the terror of the encounter with existential loneliness, and then the deepening of their sense of humanity, an awareness of love, in the deepest sense. Robyn Davidson journeyed alone 1,700 miles through the Australian desert, accompanied by four camels and a dog. As a result of her trip she found that:

I had rediscovered people in my past and come to terms with my feelings towards them. I had learnt what love was. That love wanted the best possible for those you cared for even if that excluded yourself. That before I had wanted to possess people without loving them and now I could love them and wish them the best without needing them (1980, p. 222).

Encountering our loneliness is a means of finding our unconditional regard for humanity. It is a "boundary experience," much like death awareness, which promotes self-growth. The love that stems from our loneliness encounter can be a love that comes from the richness of ourselves; in the giving of it, we renew ourselves.

On the other hand, the love that stems from our anxiety loneliness is a very needy love that drains others. We need others to define us, we need them to assure us that we are not alone (they cannot), and we try to merge with another to avoid dealing with our existential loneliness (and also responsibility). This love is the romantic kind (I will die if you leave me), and does not allow for growth. It fosters a mutually dependent relationship in which there is no growth. This is the Annie Sullivan kind of love, based on need and the vain attempt to satisfy that need. No one else can fill us up; only we can do it for ourselves.

Mature love allows us to see the uniqueness of the other, to be able to help the other for his own sake and not ours. It means being able to let go of the other. Our professional relationships need to reflect mature love so that both parties can grow.

To have a communication disorder is to encounter our isolation at some very fundamental level. We are cut off and, when communication is uncertain, we begin to experience anxiety. I always experience a mild panic reaction, for example, any time I enter a room full of deaf adults. My sign-language skills are limited to the differentiation of a *d* from *f*, which took me three beginning sign-language courses to accomplish. (I also had to promise never to reveal the name of my last teacher.) In the presence of people who are facile with sign language and for whom that is their primary means of communication, I am a severely handicapped individual. I am frightened, I hope people will not approach, and I seek to leave the situation at the first opportunity. After leaving a group of deaf people, I often think how difficult it must be for them to deal with the hearing world on an everyday basis. One could only feel isolated and frightened. What a relief it must be to encounter someone who speaks your language.

As a practicing audiologist, it became apparent to me that the underlying terror of progressive hearing loss experienced by the clients was the feeling of being cut off and isolated. The major means by which we alleviate our interpersonal loneliness is verbal communication, and when that is defective we become very disturbed. The child who would not let his mother out of sight because he could not hear her when she was in a different room in the house; the truck driver who burst into tears because he could no longer go to the bar with his cronies as he no longer heard the punch line of the jokes they told; and the wife complaining about her hearing-impaired husband who refused to go out of the house because communication was so difficult for him are quite common clinical complaints. All are loneliness experiences. The stutterer who will not use the phone, the laryngectomized adult who refuses to leave his home, and the individual with a cleft palate who avoids contact with others because his appearance and speech are so poor are all lonely people that speech pathologists will encounter. Alleviating a communication disorder then is akin to bestowing a great gift.

In a similar vein any catastrophic event that changes status isolates the individual from the familiar, throws him into a new and yet undefined identity, and forces an encounter with existential loneliness. In her book *Journey*, Suzanne Massie, the mother of a child with hemophilia, declared that:

The ostracism and isolation were almost harder to adapt to than the disease itself. More than ever we needed the help and comfort of close human contact. We needed friends. In our situation they were essential. I cannot remember a single friend who was near us in the early days of Bobby's illness. My college friends were all conducting lives of supreme normality. My catastrophe only confirmed in their minds the fact that I always had been "different." . . . It was as though we were living on an island (1973, p. 148).

She also experienced the intensity of relationship engendered by the encounter with existential loneliness.

Hemophilia has wiped out any interest or ability I might have had for superficial relationships. It sharpened my need for knowing the essentials and made me impatient with social trivialities. I wanted to know about the loves, the hates, the struggles of others (1973, p. 147).

For Helen Featherstone, loneliness is the most pervasive attribute of parents who have disabled children.

The two most prominent ingredients of a parent's loneliness are difference, his own and the child's, and isolation. The disabled child is unlike other children. He is marked in some important way, even if the difference is not immediately apparent. His mother, father, sisters and brothers live in a family that reflects that difference; their consciousness of difference makes them feel very much alone on some occasions. Failures of other people to understand their special concerns intensify the problem (1980, p. 50).

There is very little in the communication disorders literature about loneliness, yet it has to be a very common concomitant of a communication handicap. In fact I think that all communication disorders involve loneliness, and that loneliness is a distinguishing feature of communication disorder disabilities. I wonder why we ignore this issue when we can do a great deal to alleviate this special loneliness. The direct work with speech-, language-, or hearing-disabled individuals can alleviate much of the communicative isolation: for example, the empathetic thrill we feel when someone puts on their first hearing aid and "hears" again, the first time a stutterer achieves fluency, or when the aphonic finds a voice; it is just this breaking through the barriers of isolation that makes our profession rewarding.

MEANINGLESSNESS

For the existentialist there is no extrinsic meaning to the world: "We are huddled together on this orb hurtling through space in the face of cosmic indifference." This view is, or can be, very frightening because one of our most fundamental needs is a sense of direction, a purpose to our acts. Without meaning, the individual is very uncomfortable. Loss of meaning is not an uncommon cause of suicide and a frequent complaint of individuals seeking psychotherapy (Yalom, 1980). Don Juan discusses meaninglessness as follows:

"I told you once that our lot as men is to learn, for good or bad," he said. "I have learned to *see* and I tell you that nothing really matters. Now it is your turn; perhaps some day you will *see* and you will know then whether things matter or not. For me nothing matters, but perhaps for you everything will. You should know by now that a man of knowledge lives by acting; not by thinking of acting, nor by thinking about what he will think when he has finished acting. A man of knowledge chooses a path with heart and follows it; and then he looks and rejoices and laughs; and then he *sees* and knows. He knows that his life will be over altogether too soon; he knows that he as well as everybody else is not going anywhere; he knows because he sees, that nothing is more important than anything else. In other words a man of knowledge has no honor, no dignity, no family, no name, no country, but only life to be lived, and under these circumstances his only true tie to his fellow man is his controlled folly. Thus a man of knowledge endeavors, and sweats and puffs, and if one looks at him, he is just like any ordinary man, except that the folly of his life is under control. Nothing being more important than anything else; a man of knowledge chooses any act, and acts it out as if it matters to him. His controlled folly makes him say that what he does matters and makes him act as if it did, and yet he knows that it doesn't; so that when he fulfills his acts he retreats in peace, and whether his acts were good or bad or worked or didn't is in no part of his concern" (Castaneda, 1971, p. 106).

Don Juan offers the existential solution to the meaninglessness dilemma: if there is no meaning out there then we must pick one for ourselves, preferably a "path with heart." This concept can be immensely liberating because one person's meaning to the world is as good as anyone else's, and it is our existential responsibility to select meaning for ourselves. There seem to be several alternative meanings to choose from: Yalom (1980) includes (1) the traditional religious view, (2) altruism, (3) dedication to a cause, (4) creativity, (5) hedonism, and (6) self-actualization.

1. *Religious view.* The traditional Judeo–Christian model that, at least within our culture, seems to predominate holds that there is meaning and direction in our lives, that we are guided by an outside force—God—who has a plan for us, which we may not at this time understand. This view can enable the individual to accept a personal catastrophe as part of God's plan; however, as we shall see later it also leaves the door open to guilt.

2. *Altruism.* The purpose of altruism is to do good, to help others, and to leave this world a better place than when we found it. The danger in this solution is the underlying motive. If our altruism stems from anxiety loneliness we can leave people in worse shape than when we found them by rescuing them and creating dependency. Perhaps the Japanese have the best solution, they always thank the person they are helping because it gives them a chance to feel good about themselves.

3. *Dedication to a cause.* Finding a movement that is bigger than any individual and devoting oneself to it may or may not have an altruistic component; for example, we can dedicate our lives to helping the American Indians, a political party, disarmament, or saving the California condor. It is a matter of choosing one's particular cause. This solution of the meaningless issue is very much tied to responsibility assumption. It can be very tempting to allow the cause to define us—the search for a guru to give us our "cause" just leads us to evade our responsibility and if that happens it is not a good existential solution to the problem of finding meaning.

4. *Creativity.* Creativity is the wish to perpetuate ourselves in some way by leaving some legacy behind us; thus is born the impulse to write a book, have a child, or compose a symphony. This meaning fits within the generativity stage of the life cycle, which will be discussed in Chapter 3.

5. *Hedonism.* This solution to finding meaning is that the basic purpose of life is enjoyment. Hedonism is not enjoyment at the

expense of others; in fact, one can receive enjoyment from helping others. In some way hedonism may be the ultimate existential solution because it implies that there is no other purpose in life but life itself.

6. *Self-actualization*. Self-actualization is the humanistic view that I am here to become more fully what I was intended to become, to fulfill my potential.

None of these alternatives is mutually exclusive, one can adopt several or all of them; for example, one can be traditionally religious, altruistic, and dedicated to causes such as political or social movements. The existential essence of this thought, however, is that each individual must select which meaning he wishes to give to his life.

I have begun to see how important the meaning issue is in clinical practice. At its most fundamental level, having a crisis occur in life causes a crisis around meaning. The individual has to rework his position in the world as a result of a catastrophic occurrence.

Suzanne Massie, a deeply religious woman and the mother of a hemophiliac, Bobby, wrote in her book *Journey:*

And yet the need to find meaning remains. . . . Why, God, Why?

I could not consider Bobby's hemophilia punishment. When I looked at my bright-eyed child, full of energy and drive, it was unthinkable that God would meaninglessly visit His wrath upon him. . . . Could it be to teach us of suffering? The Russians saw in suffering a way to enlightenment. To them it was not a curse but a mystery with great potential for good. "Be glad Suzanne," Svetlana would say to me. "Be glad you feel deeply." "And remember," she would say, "You are a queen, because you are suffering." In the Soviet Union, a friend told me with respect, "Hemophilia is your family struggle, through it you have been able to glimpse the suffering of our Lord."

In time I came to believe. In time I became grateful that we had been given the chance to see and feel so much. And I told Bobby this; that he had been given suffering earlier than many but that, inevitably, suffering and failure come to all in life. I told him that he was fortunate to have had the chance to meet it when he was young, because those who meet it early are luckier than those whom it comes to later, when it often breaks them (1973, pp. 166–167).

A rationalization for a terrible disorder? Perhaps. A way of finding meaning from a catastrophe? Yes, and very human. Out of this tragedy has come this remarkable book and maybe that is all the meaning there needs to be to it.

Parents in particular have to find meaning because of the possibilities of guilt. Rabbi Harold Kushner was the father of a child with progeria. This very rare disorder involves rapid, premature aging so that the child dies in adolescence of old age. As a deeply religious man he had to find some justification for this tragedy. Rabbi Kushner points out that if one takes the traditional view that God is in heaven punishing the wicked and rewarding the righteous, when evil befalls us in the form of a disabled child, the individual is left with the notion that he must have sinned in some way. This view leaves parents feeling very guilty and angry at God. In his book *When Bad Things Happen to Good People*, Kushner examines the Bible and concludes that God does not cause our misery but He can be a source of solace for us if we wish. To put this in existential terms, God is there for us to use, to give meaning to the events in our lives if we choose.

EXISTENTIALISM AND THE FIELD OF COMMUNICATION DISORDERS

The existential message for us as professionals is quite clear and very meaningful. We are humans and we too must come to grips with these existential issues. If we fail to deal with issues around our own death we will take no risks. Responsibility evasion will lead to no growth. If we avoid our loneliness we will not find mature love. Until we resolve for ourselves the meaning crisis, we will lack direction and commitment. All of these existential givens impinge directly on our ability to function effectively as clinicians and, until we resolve them for ourselves, we will be limited in our effectiveness.

Existential issues abound within our clinical interactions. Since I have discovered the vocabulary and notions of the existentialists, I feel the excitement of the Molière character who discovers that he has been speaking prose all his life. The existential issues have been there all along, it is a matter of seeing them. Yalom (1980) has commented that psychiatrists do not deal with these issues because they have not resolved them for themselves. I think that is partly true for me, but I have also needed the theoretical framework in order to see the client behavior.

For example, within a parent group session the following things happened:

A parent was knocked down by a car before the session (not seriously injured).
A participant was feeling very lonely and cut off because she was far from home.
A parent was worried because her grandmother was undergoing a serious operation.
During the course of the meeting a mother cried, "Life is not fair."

All of these events could and did at some point lead to a discussion around an existential issue. As with any clinical tool, it is handy to have this frame of reference available, and it can be used with profit to allow the clinician to understand the deeper issues that our clients are grappling with.

The encounters with death, either real or symbolic, as experienced by many of the clients we encounter, can lead them to an examination of their life priorities. The speech and hearing clinician must be sensitive to these changing priorities and help the person let go of old self-images. The stroke victim, for example, will have to deal with the same death issues as the cancer patients cited earlier in this chapter. In addition, he will be cut off from communicating many of these thoughts. The speech clinician can be the vital link to his new reality.

Responsibility assumption is fundamental to any of the changes we are hoping to accomplish with the communicatively disordered. The therapist must be very sensitive to the rescue syndrome and must not take responsibility away from the clients. We must build in therapeutic techniques that allow and encourage an inner locus of control to develop. When the client develops an inner locus of control, carryover is no longer a problem. Once a client assumes responsibility for his speech behavior, we have little else to teach him.

The professional can do much to eliminate or reduce the interpersonal loneliness that is the concomitant of a communication disorder or of any catastrophic change. The clinician can help most to alleviate loneliness by careful empathetic listening. When we can hear and respond to the "faint knocking" of the lonely, frightened person, then a beautiful energy—love—flows between us. Our presence in their world and our shared moments are marvelous gifts we can bring to others. In the long run, that is all we ever have.

We can also organize groups in which parents can meet other parents who have similar problems. A special relationship is established among parents that transcends any parent-professional relationship. There is the rapport and instant understanding that occurs among people who "have been there." Similarly, groups of stutterers, hearing-impaired adults, or aphasics (especially their families) benefit from contact. The speech pathologist/audiologist can provide the means for them to meet, and can facilitate their growth through the group interaction. This subject will be discussed further in Chapter 5.

I often see parents undergoing the crisis of meaning much as Rabbi Kushner and Mrs. Massie did in the examples cited earlier. The issue has important clinical implications. Usually out of this meaning crisis comes a dedication to a cause—for example, parents who become teachers of the deaf or very active in state or national organizations—which can be a very wholesome direction of parental energies. I also see a great deal of altruism that flows to and from the parents. I never pity these parents; I know that this crisis gives them a chance to find a new meaning for themselves and to lead a richer life. Because it is a meaning that they have selected with thought for themselves, it is almost invariably a "path with heart."

And how about the speech pathologist? For Van Riper, the grand old man of our profession, "the author [Van Riper] has been privileged to spend his life seeking to reduce, prevent and heal that special kind of human misery found in defective speech and it has a given him a sense of meaningfulness he hungers to share" (1972, p. 2).

And that might have to suffice for all of us in this profession.

B I B L I O G R A P H Y

ASHA interview: Geri Jewell. *ASHA* 25:18, 1983.

Bodner, B., and Johns, J. Personality and hearing impairment: A study in locus of control. *Volta Rev.* 79:362, 1977.

Castaneda, C. *A Separate Reality.* New York: Simon & Schuster, 1971.

Castaneda, C. *Journey to Ixacton.* New York: Simon & Schuster, 1972.

Davidson, R. *Tracks.* London: Butler & Tanner, 1980.

Dowaliby, F., Burke, N., and McKee, B. A comparison of hearing impaired and normally hearing students on locus of control, people orientation, and study habits and attitudes. *Am. Ann. Deaf* 128:53, 1983.

Featherstone, H. *A Difference in the Family.* New York: Basic Books, 1980.

Fromm, E. *Escape from Freedom.* New York: Holt, Rinehart & Winston, 1941.

Hallahan, P. P., Gasar, A. H., Cohen, S. B., and Tarver, S. C. Selective attention and locus of control in learning disabled and normal children. *J. Learning Disord.* 11:47, 1978.

Hornyak, A. The rescue game and the speech-language pathologist, *ASHA* 22:86, 1980.

Kübler-Ross, E. *On Death and Dying.* New York: Macmillan, 1969.

Kushner, H. *When Bad Things Happen to Good People.* New York: Avon Books, 1983.

Land, S. L., and Vineberg, S. E. Locus of control in blind children. *Except. Child.* 31:257, 1965.

Lash, J. V. *Helen and Teacher.* New York: Delacorte, 1980.

Massie, R., and Massie, S. *Journey.* New York: Knopf, 1973.

Mitford, J. *The American Way of Death.* New York: Simon & Schuster, 1963.

Moustakes, C. *Loneliness.* Englewood Cliffs, N.J.: Prentice-Hall, 1961.

Munro, J., and Bach, T. Effect of time limited counseling on client change. *J. Counseling Psychol.* 22:395, 1975.

Shirlberg, L., Diabless, D., Carlson, K., Filley, F., Kwiatkowski, J., and Smith, M. Personality characteristics, academic performance and clinical competence in communication disorders majors. *ASHA* 19:311, 1977.

Shlien, J., Mosak, H., and Dreikors, R. Effects of time limits: A comparison of two psychotherapies. *J. Counseling Psychol.* 9:31, 1962.

Tanner, D. C. Loss and grief: Implications for the speech language pathologists and audiologists. *ASHA* 22:916, 1980.

Van Riper, C. *Speech Correction* (5th ed.). Englewood Cliffs, N.J.: Prentice-Hall, 1972.

Webster, M. *Hear here. Newsletter of the Canadian Speech and Hearing Association* 6:235, 1982.

White, K. Defining and prioritizing the personal and social competence needed by hearing impaired students. *Volta Rev.* 84:266, 1982.

Wright, D. *Deafness.* New York: Stein & Day, 1969.

Yalom, I. *Existential Psychotherapy.* New York: Basic Books, 1980.

CHAPTER 3

ERIKSON LIFE CYCLE

AND RELATIONSHIP

Among the pantheon of my personal gurus, Erik Erikson rates highly. The son of a Jewish mother, a Danish father, and a Jewish stepfather, he came of age in Germany during the rise of Hitler. As a youth he was an itinerant artist, a euphemism for a young man without much direction. He was employed as a tutor in a family that was friendly with Freud. Anna Freud, trained as an elementary school teacher, became interested in applying psychoanalytic therapy—developed by her father—to the raising of children, and became involved with the family that Erikson was tutoring. He became swept up in the psychoanalytic movement and entered psychoanalysis (which was a requirement for anyone seeking to become a psychoanalyst) with Anna Freud. Erikson finished his psychoanalytic training in 1933 and, because of the deteriorating conditions in Germany and his Jewish family connections, emigrated with his family to the United States. He worked in Boston for several years as a child analyst, one of the first analysts in the United States to specialize in children.

Erikson subsequently moved to the west coast and studied child-raising practices of the Sioux and Yurok tribes as well as the children enrolled at the Institute of Child Welfare in California. He became quite interested in how culture shapes personality and, with the eye of a painter and the training of a clinician, he observed the evolution of the life cycle from infancy to death. Among Erikson's many works, probably the most outstanding is his book *Childhood and Society* (1950) in which he first delineated his observation of the life cycle. (Readers interested in further pursuing the life and work of Erikson are referred to the excellent biography written by Robert Coles.)

This frequently used and quoted model of the life cycle—often called the "eight stages of man"—is an immensely useful way to look at the developing ego qualities in the child and adult, which emerge from critical periods of development. Erikson feels that each successive stage has a special relationship to a basic element of society because the life cycle and our institutions have evolved together. Each stage of ego development or "crisis" needs to be resolved, at least partially, before one can successfully move on to the next stage. It is possible to think of each stage as a continuum in which the child establishes that ego development feature. This is a hierarchical structure in which each developmental issue is present in the previous stage and is worked out further in subsequent stages. Each stage is presented as a duality and the usual outcome is a balance between the two extremes.

TRUST VS. MISTRUST

At this first stage the infant must come to recognize that the world is basically a safe place—that her needs are going to be met and that there is some consistency and order to the world. In order to feel trust, the world must be predictable and the people who inhabit that world (mainly the primary caretaker) must be trustworthy and responsive to the child's needs in predictable and positive ways. Failure to develop this basic trust leads to the development of the severest forms of infantile schizophrenia.

AUTONOMY VS. SHAME AND DOUBT

During this stage the child develops a sense of personal power, of having some control over the world. This begins as she establishes some control, both motor and mental, over self. As speech and language develop the child can make her wants known and begin to control others. Unfortunately for adults, autonomy is frequently interpreted as a negative reaction to the desires of the parents (thus is born the "terrible twos"). The task of the parents is to help the child develop a sense of autonomy with a benign conscience. If the child is controlled by shame, this tends to lead to an adult who governs by the letter of the law rather than the spirit, and to the development of compulsive behavior.

INITIATIVE VS. GUILT

In this stage the child learns to be assertive, to take risks. The normal child moves into the larger adult society in an intrusive manner characterized by vigorous movements, and by occasional aggressiveness (especially toward siblings). There is also an insatiable curiosity manifested by the asking of endless questions. The task of the parents is to allow the child movement into the adult world without clamping down too much so as to limit initiative. Too many restrictions by the parents cause the child to develop a highly constricted conscience based on guilt, which limits the child's willingness to risk. The psychopathology at this stage leads to an adult who exhibits hysterical denial, overconstricts herself to the point of self-obliteration, or develops a great many psychosomatic diseases.

INDUSTRY VS. INFERIORITY

This stage coincides with the so-called latency period although when one examines what occurs during this stage, it is clear that *latency* is a misnomer. The child, equipped with a sense of trust in the world and with some trust in self because she has been allowed to develop autonomy and initiative, usually is now ready to learn formal skills. Society accommodates by providing the school in its many manifestations; here she learns the technological fundamentals of the society. She learns the adult tools that will be necessary in order to assume adulthood. The danger to the child at this stage is that she may not develop a sense of adequacy either through the failure of the family to prepare the child for school or the failure of the school to capitalize on the child's emerging abilities. An adult who has had difficulty at the industry level develops feelings of inadequacy compared with her peer group.

IDENTITY VS. ROLE CONFUSION

Erikson's recognition of the adolescent experience as predominantly an issue of identity has received a great deal of attention and confirmation from developmental psychologists. The adolescent's task is to establish independence and freedom from the family and then, in the latter stages of adolescence, to establish a social role for herself. Identity is really accomplished through life experiences. As we encounter situations in which we have some success and some failure, we learn more about ourselves and we get a more rounded picture of ourselves. The adolescent has a limited life experience and so generally models herself after a significant adult. This adult can be a character in a play or a movie. I think many adolescents, for example, decided to become teachers of the deaf after seeing the movie *The Miracle Worker*. In fact I always ask students in my classes how they became interested in becoming speech therapists or teachers of the deaf. In my first classes almost all students said they entered the profession because they were exposed to deafness via a deaf relative or a deaf friend. More recently the classes, while still having a large number of students who were exposed early to deafness, also have a large minority who were exposed through media: government-sponsored advertising, plays and movies that have featured the handicapped, or programs arranged in the elementary schools to sensitize students to the handicapped.

The adolescent also must establish identity in relationship to the same-sex parent and this usually appears as a rejection of parental values. As Erikson (1950) so charmingly puts it, the adolescents often "must artificially appoint perfectly well meaning people to play the roles of adversaries." How sensitively the parent is able to handle the conflict, while maintaining a flexibility and above all else a sense of humor, will determine the adolescent's ability both to acquire a good sense of self and to select a reasonably suitable occupational goal. In any event, "identity" will have to be reworked in adulthood as one comes into possession of more and more data about self. In one sense life is a succession of "identity crises" as we move through the life cycle and are forced to discard old concepts of ourselves to acquire the new.

INTIMACY VS. ISOLATION

Erikson was one of the first child analysts to recognize that the life cycle did not cease at adolescence but continued on into adulthood. Adulthood is not static but fraught with crises. As a child I often thought that when I was 30 I would "have it all together." I now recognize that growth is a continuous process: at times there are plateaus and at other times there are "break-up" periods. I now think that the times when we have it all together are just interludes to be enjoyed and savored.

The young adult is now a free and self-governing individual; her task is to establish new ties to the world, free of the family relationships. These new ties will involve the establishment of new primary relationships and an occupation. Those adults who have a fragile sense of identity dare not enter into intimate relationships for fear of losing self, while those individuals who have little sense of self try to fuse with another and establish their identity through the other person. In a truly intimate, loving relationship both parties can and do maintain their separate identities. The young adult must find this balance—not an easy task.

Work also involves a fusion in which one must try to maintain a separate identity while feeling a part of the institution. Individuals with fragile egos become fearful of being swallowed by the institution and fail to commit themselves, while individuals with little personal sense of identity will tend to overcommit themselves and merge their personal identity with their work identity. Neither solution is healthy, and the failure to solve the intimacy crisis leads to a deep sense of isolation and alienation.

GENERATIVITY VS. STAGNATION

This stage involves the need to ensure the existence of the species either by literally becoming a parent or by sharing knowledge and skills with the young. It is the life cycle stage that is characterized by productivity and creativity. This is the stage of altruism whereby the adult foregoes her own personal needs to care for others. Generativity does not necessarily mean becoming a parent. One can figuratively instruct or care for future generations through work or charity. Mature humans, according to Erikson, need to instruct and teach. Thus is born the impulse to become a parent, write a book, compose a symphony, and so on.

The mere fact that one becomes a parent does not ensure that one has arrived at generativity. Some parents who have not resolved earlier issues around intimacy and identity are not able to give. They are still very self-absorbed and narcissistic as one would expect at an earlier stage of ego development. In a similar vein, one's work can be long and strenuous but not very productive. Generativity enriches the individual as well as society; when such enrichment fails to take place, the individual stagnates.

EGO INTEGRITY VS. DESPAIR

For the aging or aged adult who has successfully negotiated the previous seven stages, this is the age of wisdom and detachment. It is the ability to see human problems in their entirety in the face of approaching death. One is able to love on a species-wide basis in the deepest sense. The mature elderly continue to grow and to adjust. The mature adult with ego integrity does not fear death, she recognizes it as an integral part of the life cycle. Growing old does not guarantee that one will grow wise. There are elderly adults who fear death, who feel that life is now too short for them to engage in any new endeavor, and who are mired in despair.

LIFE CYCLE AND
COMMUNICATION DISORDERS

Use of the Erikson life cycle model in the field of communication disorders has not been extensive. I have found only one detailed use of it. Schlessinger and Meadow (1971), in their study of deafness and mental health, used the Erikson model as a theory for explaining the discrepancy between the normal potential and the relatively poor achievement of the deaf person. Using their clinical experience, they have found the developmental framework provided by the life cycle model valuable in looking at the deaf child. It appears that at each life cycle stage the deaf child has a more formidable task resolving that particular crisis than does the normally hearing child. There has, however, been no rigorous scientific investigation of how deafness affects the life cycle.

One might presume, for example, that the development of basic trust may be impaired because of the delays and uncertainties in diagnosing the deafness and the consequent anxiety in the parents. The parental grief reaction, which involves a great deal of anger and sorrow, also suggests that the deaf child may not receive the consistency of parental care and responsiveness, which is vital to the development of trust. From the deaf infant's point of view while undergoing diagnosis the world must seem a very frightening place with many strangers and many unexplained parental absences.

The lack of clear communication can limit the development of autonomy and initiative in a deaf child. Parents, for example, cannot explain why a rule is imposed nor can the child ask the necessary questions to find out about her world. Parents tend to limit their child physically because of the deafness and the fear that the child may not hear if called. There is also a high parental anxiety, which is reflected in the attitude that "I let something bad happen to you once and I'm not about to let something bad happen to you again."

At the competency level the deaf child is again limited by the poor communication skills and the overprotection of teachers and parents. Much of our skill acquisition is dependent on explanation. Teacher expectation of deaf children as "low achievers" may also limit the competency of the deaf child who tends to internalize this judgment of the significant adults in her world.

Identity problems are particularly acute in the deaf child of hearing parents. In addition to the normal struggle to establish self, the deaf child has an apparent choice between the "hearing world" and the "deaf world." Her problems are compounded if she has been raised orally based on a denial of deafness such that there is no hearing-impaired peer group to relate to nor any significant deaf adults to use as a role model.

Schlessinger and Meadow (1971) have observed that the young deaf people whom they have seen have been poorly equipped by the schools for the deaf for their introduction into the adult world. According to them the young adult deaf person is not prepared for the intangible rules of the hearing society and frequently regresses to a more dependent status, much to the chagrin of teachers and parents. It is also hard for the young deaf adults to develop a sense of generativity because of society's discrimination against the deaf. Love and work become very difficult under such conditions.

Almost nothing is known about the aged deaf—this is largely an unexplored area of investigation. One may presume that with the increased difficulty that they experience at each life cycle level, few deaf people achieve ego integrity or if they do, they must travel a different route, one that is harder and more circuitous than that of the hearing population.

It would be very interesting to use the Erikson model on other disabled populations to see how they are affected; to my knowledge this has not been done.

LIFE CYCLE AND RELATIONSHIP BUILDING

I have found the life cycle model to be a very useful way of looking at the development of a healthy counseling relationship, which is critical for growth. I find I can use this model at times to diagnose relationships that do not seem to be working—to find where I need to get back to in order to have a more fruitful relationship. It helps to understand how to build a relationship as there is also a hierarchical function to relationship-building similar to that in the life cycle model in which each stage that is worked on has its origins in previous stages and is worked out further in later stages.

TRUST

Trust is the bedrock of a healthy relationship. Unfortunately, many professional relationships are not built on trust, and there can be no growth in relationships unless trust is present. There are three basic elements to building trust: caring, consistency, and credibility.

Caring is conveyed to the client in any number of ways, not the least of which is by active and sensitive listening. Kopp, a psychotherapist, writes:

> My first task was the creation of an atmosphere of trust within which we could enter into a therapeutic alliance.
>
> I begin by listening carefully to what a new patient has to say and to how it is said. I do not yet listen for the underlying dynamics that contribute to the patient's unhappiness. At the beginning, I am only trying to discover how it must feel to be that particular patient. For a while I do little more than try to formulate how the patient feels and to reflect those feelings back to the patient. It is enough that she finds that I am trying to understand how she experiences her life and that I help her to clarify her feelings without judging them (1978, p. 81).

The key to the notion of trust-building is nonjudgmental listening. If someone is willing to try to hear my fears and my concerns and responds to my feelings without telling me that I "shouldn't feel that way," then I can be more open and trusting. Joysa Post, a speech-language pathologist who had a cerebrovascular accident and subsequently was aphasic, found that the quality she responded to the most in the clinicians who worked with her was caring. She needed a clinician "who cared and was interested in me as a person" (1983).

Trust develops when I believe that the people I am dealing with are reliable. This again is shown by the very simple things that clinicians can do. I start meetings on time and always end them when we have agreed to end them. If I cannot be at a meeting, I warn the clients ahead of time. If I have misrepresented issues or erred in some way, I apologize and correct the error. I try to be transparent about my feelings and my concerns. I also never tell clients anything that I cannot verify.

We are granted credibility by virtue of title in the initial stages of relationship. We give trust to someone who bears the title "Doctor" (especially if she wears a white coat). Over time, however, credibility has to be earned. In part we earn it by what we know and how we convey it. The information given by the professional early in diagnosis is seldom retained by the clients because affect is so high. What is being worked on without either party being aware of it is the establishment of credibility. I will trust a professional if I think she knows her field even if at that point I do not have a sufficient corpus of stored information to evaluate the information being provided.

There are also all the intangibles of credibility establishment, which are conveyed to others by how I conduct myself, if I seem to be in control of myself, and if I share my information. Oddly enough I have found that I do not lose credibility, in fact I gain it, when I am willing to tell clients that I do not know something. They are then willing to trust the other information that I provide. If I am willing to tag something as unknown by me, it gives them the confidence to believe what I say is known. (Of course, there are times when what I think is "known" is not a fact—too many of these assumptions and I lose all credibility. It is my professional responsibility to keep my information up to date.)

One of the surest ways to lose credibility is by reassurance. While the people we are dealing with frequently seek reassurance, when we give it we also diminish ourselves. When we tell people that it will be okay in order to help make them feel better, they also know that we cannot *know* that it will be better, and we lose credibility. I am always suspicious of anyone who seems to be telling me what I want to hear: at one level it is validating, at another, though, I lose trust in what the person is telling me.

A U T O N O M Y

Autonomy in a relationship is the feeling that I can control what goes on, that I can make things happen that I perceive are in my best interests. Autonomy is always established in relationship to someone else; it is a bouncing-off that requires some form of negotiation with someone else, usually someone who is perceived as being more powerful.

Often the powerful other is the professional. How much autonomy do we allow in therapy? My observation of most therapy is that very little autonomy is granted to the client. I think this comes about as a result of the "lesson plan syndrome." Students in training are expected to enter therapy with a specific plan and goals. This gives the therapist, especially the insecure beginning therapist, control of the situation. More experienced therapists will be flexible and modify a plan depending on the client. How many therapists, I wonder, develop the lesson plans in conjunction with the specific client, where both will sit down and decide the agenda for that meeting. Autonomy can be encouraged in such little ways, for example, by the audiologist asking the client after a diagnostic evaluation, "What do you need to know?" rather than delivering a set speech and making all the decisions regarding the kind of information needed.

The professional gets worried in giving autonomy to the client on two counts, the first of which is the time element. When there is a waiting room full of patients it is much quicker to give the set speech and send the client out the door. The expeditious solution is usually the least efficient on a long-term basis, because the set speech is rarely retained and the client will return with the same lack of knowledge.

Second, the professional is worried that "they might not ask the right questions." In the context of an establishment of a counseling relationship, there are no wrong questions. Generally, if the client does not ask the question, she is not ready to hear the answer and the information provided is seldom digested. People will learn just what they are ready to learn and absorb. The best indication of readiness is the question: gratuitous information usually serves to increase confusion and is rarely helpful. There are times when it is appropriate for the professional to provide information without being asked. When this device is successful, it is generally because we have responded to the unasked question, which requires first sensitive listening.

INITIATIVE

Initiative is an element of relationships that is very closely related to autonomy. Initiative is the positive side of autonomy. Autonomy is usually established by the "no" in relationship to the powerful other and in some ways is easier than the initiative because we do not have to take responsibility for our behavior. It is much easier to know what you do not want than to take the responsibility for getting what you do want. Initiative is fostered by the professional leaving spaces—teaching by creating vacuums. If I do not take total responsibility for what is going on, then the other person in the relationship has to act. It may seem damaging to the ego, but the less I do, the more the other person learns in the relationship. We are going to have to change some of the definitions of professional responsibility. So often the professional must "do" in order to satisfy the job description and the supervisors. Listening and responding are not always seen by either the therapist or the supervisor as being effective professional behavior. We need to change this attitude. Professionals are going to have to learn to be comfortable with silences and with "not doing" so as to create spaces in which the client can act and learn.

There are some dangers in this approach to fostering initiative. For one, we will violate the client's expectation of what a professional should do. ("Why am I paying you?") This violation will generate anger, which may or may not surface, that if not dealt with, can distort the relationship. The anger itself is a marvelous spur to taking initiative on the client's part if the clinician can sensitively handle it. Second, if we do not act we may lose credibility; there is a thin line that the professional must very delicately tread. The difference for me is in being responsible *to* (or responsive *to*) the clients rather than being responsible *for* them. Although I try to do 50 percent of the work and invite the other person to do her 50 percent, it is often hard to locate the therapeutic equator of responsibility.

Autonomy and initiative are attributes that are especially important for parents of handicapped children to develop. They will need these traits in devising educational plans for their children in conjunction with the public school professionals. It is so easy for the parents to be intimidated by the confrontation with professionals. By now, it should also be clear to the reader that initiative and autonomy are "loci of control" issues. Inner locus of control is obtained through the development of initiative and autonomy.

INDUSTRY

Industry is the relationship level in which most professionals seem to relate to their clients. There is clearly a task to be accomplished, a communication disorder to be overcome, a deaf child to be educated, a hearing aid to be obtained. Unfortunately, most professionals are so content- or problem-centered that they ignore the trust, autonomy, and initiative issues. The professional anxiety to alleviate the problem gets in the way of the establishment of the necessary precursors to effective joint work. The therapeutic alliance is not established and the professionals do much more than their 50 percent and then proceed to complain about lack of client motivation.

Learning is obtained by any of three routes: by being told (lecture), by seeing (demonstration), and by doing. The most lasting way of learning is by doing. Unfortunately, for parent groups in particular, the professionals seem to use the lecture as the primary learning vehicle. Many parent discussion groups are really lectures provided by the professional on some topic that may or may not be selected by the parent group. A lecture is a very inefficient way to teach because it assumes incorrectly that your audience is homogeneous in knowledge. The degree to which the learners have developed some trust will be reflected in their willingness to ask questions and take some initiative for their own learning. It is often difficult to get a parent group to ask questions after a lecture because there is a low level of trust in the group.

The demonstration as a teaching device is very tricky. If it is not used sensitively then it can de-skill (strip) the learner of feelings of competency. I have seen this occur repeatedly in itinerant therapy programs in which I have worked with both the teachers and the parents of young deaf children. In this program the teacher had to travel several hours to get to the parents' home; thus she had only a limited time to spend with the child. The teacher brought in the child's favorite toy and gave a surefire, brilliant lesson. The child was generally very eager to see the teacher as she only came once a week and always had a new toy to play with. The lesson almost invariably went well and the therapist would then tell the parent to continue working on this lesson during the week. When the parent tried to do the lesson by imitating what she had seen the therapist do, however, she invariably failed. The failure occurred for a variety of reasons: the child was too familiar with the parent and resented parent as teacher; the parent had many emotional issues about the child and often was not able to see the child clearly; and the parent was probably not very competent (why should she be?), which is why she was in the program in the first place. In itinerant programs of this sort the parent is almost always programmed for failure, and thus begins to feel even more incompetent.

My own bias about itinerant programs is that they should be all parent-centered. I think that the teacher needs to see the parent as the recipient of her teaching and should only rarely work directly with the child.

A similar loss of competency can occur when the supervisor demonstrates to the student clinician a more effective way to establish the desired behavior in a client. This demonstration is usually done easily and effortlessly by the supervisor and leaves the student feeling totally incompetent. The supervisor who goes to a conference and observes a master clinician at work may also feel incompetent. Demonstration, if not done sensitively, can have the opposite of the intended effect and leave the learner in worse shape. This is not to say demonstration does not have a place in teaching; it can be a very valuable tool when there is enough trust in the relationship and when the learner already has established some self-esteem.

"Doing" is by far the most efficient way to learn, especially if one has a sensitive supervisor-teacher observing. Doing requires the highest degree of trust, for no one likes to appear incompetent and the learner, by definition, is supposed to be incompetent. In order to learn, the student must be willing to reveal her areas of ignorance to the teacher. Unfortunately, most educational programs reward competency and penalize ignorance; therefore, students learn to try and please the teacher by guessing what is in the teacher's head and by trying to appear competent when they are not.

Holt (1964) noticed that elementary school children, when given the task of trying to guess a number, would be disturbed by a "no" answer despite the fact that they gained as much information from a "no" answer as they did from a "yes." He concluded that one of the reasons children fail is because they are afraid of failure. No initiative can be taken unless there is a willingness to be wrong. In order for effective learning to take place, we must remove all penalty for failure and we must encourage mistakes (to put that another way, we must encourage learners to take risks). I have learned far more from my mistakes than I have from my successes. The failure tells me where my limit is and where I need to learn more. My successes, while gratifying, reflect skills that I have already mastered and no longer need to learn.

The unconditional regard, the caring that I convey to the learners, allows them to take risks. In short, there must be trust present for skills to be taught and learned. Each of these techniques of lecturing, demonstrating, and doing has a value in learning and, in a particular time and place, each one may be appropriate. As we shall see in the next chapter, timing is all-important.

IDENTITY

Identity is very much role-dependent; that is, how I define myself and how others define me will determine my behavior to a large degree. It is a function of the expectations that I and others have for that particular role. It is very easy to become role-bound.

For example, the role of the "parent" has a connotation of someone who is not really involved in the educational or therapeutic process of the child. I remember once waiting outside my child's school to pick her up after an extracurricular activity. The principal, who did not know me, was concerned about a man lurking near the school. He asked me who I was and I responded, "I am *just* a parent." Without skipping a beat and for which I will be eternally grateful he responded, "What do you mean, *just* a parent?" We discussed that issue at length. Parents, as they usually define themselves in relationship to the school, are an appendage of their child, someone who provides transportation, the lunch money, and attends P.T.A. meetings to be told things about their child. They are always on the periphery of things and not really important to the learning process that is taking place in the school, which is essentially between teacher and child.

The role of "patient" also has a connotation of passivity, which is precisely why I have used the word *client* rather than *patient* throughout this text. The whole process of becoming a patient involves losing individuality. A patient goes to the doctor, receives a prescription, and follows it in order to get well. In a hospital setting, the patient is expected to be a very passive part of the process while all the professionals "operate." When patients refuse to cooperate—that is, conform to the role expectation—the doctors and nurses are immensely disturbed.

Martha Lear's book *Heartsounds* gives a remarkable view of the patient process from someone who had seen it from a physician's perspective. Her husband Hal Lear, a physician, found that when he became a heart patient the attending physicians stopped listening to him and began treating him as a disease rather than as a person. His first act in recovering from his heart attack was to stop wearing the hospital johnny coat to recover some of his personhood.

The holistic health movement, which seems to be gaining more respect these days, puts the patients at the center of the healing process and requires them to take some responsibility for the course of therapy. I hope that this trend will continue in medical practice.

Probably the most role-bound indiviudal in the therapeutic process is the professional. She is usually defined as the person who has the knowledge and the skill to make the other person better; therefore, the professional has the responsibility for making things happen, in short for being "smart" and having the answers. Professionals are expected to write prescriptions and give advice. The manner of dress is usually very narrowly prescribed (in some settings it has to be a white coat) and the terms of address are carefully spelled out—usually with a formality that keeps a patient-therapist distance. Most of this self-protective behavior is taught at the training level and is readily consumed by the student clinician. A fully defined role is a means of gaining security: if one knows exactly what is expected, then one can conform to those expectations and behave appropriately. The price one pays for this security is a rigidity in behavior that may very well limit growth. In fact, very often the traditional patient-therapist relationship has many features that limit the development of a healthy relationship. In particular, the traditional relationship fails in the responsibility assumption area, or the locus of control seems to be external to the patient and in the hands of the therapist.

In the wholesome counseling relationship, where there are high levels of trust, where both parties are free to take initiatives and have retained their autonomy, and where there are no specific role definitions, it might be very hard for the casual observer to decide who is the professional and who is the patient.

INTIMACY

Intimacy is very much tied to trust. When a high level of trust exists in a relationship, we can risk being open. Openness leads to a sense of caring and closeness. Intimacy also involves risk, and the fear of intimacy often manifests itself by self-defeating behavior, which is personally distancing.

In a counseling relationship both parties need to feel that they can say anything—not everything. Only what is important between them needs to be discussed and revealed. I do not have to disclose my bank balance in order to be intimate; however, when appropriate, I do need to relate—either verbally or nonverbally—how I feel about you. There is surety in knowing how the other person in a relationship is feeling. Intimacy also involves negative feelings. A great deal of trust is required before I can reveal to you that I am angry at you. Professionals who are role-bound often feel that they do not have the right to be angry at clients. This attitude severely limits intimacy because no true intimacy is possible unless the full range of feelings that exist in a relationship can be expressed.

Intimacy carries with it the possibility of pain. As I become more caring and closer to people, I also leave myself vulnerable to loss when the relationship ends. Because of the anticipated pain of separation, many people limit their closeness. The price of this solution is an interpersonal loneliness. Here again each of us must make a personal choice and resolve the interpersonal dilemma for ourselves. Teaching—and by extension, clinical work—is a very painful profession because many of our relationships are clearly limited in duration. The temptation by the professional to limit intimacy and pain is therefore very great, which means that we do not develop relationships that have maximum growth possibilities. I have found that when I limit risks, I also limit gains; hence, I have chosen to develop close relationships. The price I pay in June when both students and parents depart is well worth the joy I have experienced during the semester. No relationships are permanent; therefore, I want to and choose to extract the most from each relationship that I have.

GENERATIVITY

Generativity becomes the outward manifestation of the skills learned during the industry phase. Now the client can go beyond the therapeutic relationship and demonstrate and develop increased skills in other life relationships. This becomes the therapeutic carry-over issue.

Out of the successful therapeutic relationship should also come the impulse toward altruism—toward making things better for others. It is no accident that many of our speech pathologists were themselves at one time recipients of therapy. While this might also reflect an identity issue, very often it is a reflection of the desire to give others something of value that has been received. This is the noblest human drive.

I have watched parents go through the grieving process; they generally tend to progress from concern about themselves to concern about their child and finally, to concern about all deaf children. Parents are potentially a major resource for change, and the desire to help others can be channeled by the clinician to provide huge benefits to the community. Parents can and do become very active in promoting legislation and prodding bureaucrats into doing the things that they should be doing. This very fruitful energy arises from a healthy therapeutic relationship that grows into the generativity or productivity stage. How this energy is directed is determined in part by how the individual resolves the crisis around the existential issues of meaning.

I N T E G R I T Y

Integrity is the terminal phase of the relationship. Our job as therapists and teacher is to do ourselves out of our job, to no longer be needed. We are not doing our job well if we cannot let go of the clients we are serving, and, while this is painful, termination needs to be recognized as a necessary part of the therapeutic cycle.

Because of my own death avoidance, I once tried to keep termination discussion in my relationships to an absolute minimum. I see now that this was a mistake. There is a need to "close up shop," to take a detached view of the relationship and to process the experience. There is a need to bring the relationship to a closure, to explain why I did or did not do certain things, to talk about previously concealed feelings, and to express the often latent feelings of appreciation. I usually feel a sense of sadness at this time and a sense of loss. I also think about the new relationships that will be starting in the fall, and I feel a momentary sense of despair at having to start the process over again. I wonder if the new relationships will be as satisfying. I also feel some excitement at the prospect of encountering new people and learning something more about myself.

MODELS AS CLINICAL TOOLS

Models can be very dangerous if taken literally by the unwary reader because they are a simplification of a very complex process. It might seem from reading this chapter that relationship-building proceeds smoothly through the eight outlined stages and if a relationship is stuck then all one has to do is diagnose the trouble by going back to the sticking point. In practice this is not so simple; relationship-building is at best a sloppy process with different stages being worked on at different times, not necessarily sequentially. At times some issues are only partially worked out and then returned to and very often several stages are being worked on simultaneously.

Models become clinically valuable as conceptualizations; they enable us to talk about very complex phenomena by giving us a vocabulary. The reader must always bear in mind that the model is a simplification and not the event—it is but a particular abstraction of an event.

I have found the existential model and the Erikson life cycle model to be particularly helpful clinically. They complement one another nicely. The existential view focuses on current behavior that seems to be universal, whereas the Erikson model gives a developmental perspective within our culture. There are large areas of overlap between them, for example, the Erikson stages of autonomy and initiative relate to the existential issue of responsibility assumption; identity and productivity are intricately related to the meaning issue; trust and intimacy are very much part of the loneliness experience; and of course, death is part and parcel of the ego integrity stage.

Despite the overlap, these models give us somewhat different views of human beings, and we can use whichever conceptualization seems most appropriate for describing a particular behavior. There is no "right" view of human behavior, only a variety of ways to interpret a particular facet of behavior.

In the next chapters we will look at some other ways of viewing behavior with an eye toward clinical applications.

BIBLIOGRAPHY

Coles, R. *Erik H. Erikson: The Growth of His Work.* Boston: Little, Brown, 1970.

Erikson, E. H. *Childhood and Society.* New York: Norton, 1950, 1963 (2nd ed.).

Holt, J. *How Children Fail.* New York: Dell, 1964.

Kopp, S. *An End to Innocence.* New York: Bantam, 1978.

Lear, M. *Heartsounds.* New York: Simon & Schuster, 1980.

Post, J. I'd rather tell a story than be one. *ASHA* 25:22, 1983.

Schlessinger, H., and Meadow, K. *Deafness and Mental Health: A Developmental Approach.* Research grant #14-P-55270/9-03 (RD 2835-S). U.S. Department of Health, Education and Welfare, 1971.

CHAPTER 4

THE THEORY

AND PRACTICE OF

COUNSELING

The general theory that an individual holds about counseling is a reflection of his attitudes about humans and how they learn, change, and grow. Theory in this context becomes synonymous with "point of view"; and that in turn reflects how the counselor views client behavior. The problem with theory is that it quickly can become dogma and thus severely limits the response of the counselor. I think that counselors must choose a particular way of approaching clients and must be willing to be flexible depending on the context of the client-clinician relationship.

Contemporary counseling theory can be divided into five schools, each with a particular approach and with considerable overlap among the various schools.

1. *Psychoanalytic.* Some of the basic assumptions of the psychoanalytic approach are that current human behavior is deter-

mined by the conflict between instinctual drives and social restrictions. The therapist, through a variety of techniques, helps
the patient uncover unconscious material that is determining the
current maladjusted behavior. By gaining insight, which is
thought to be crucial to any change, into the causes of his current behavior, the patient is then presumably able to make the
necessary changes. The psychoanalytic approach is essentially a
medical model with a sick patient coming to the doctor to be
cured.

2. *Existentialism.* As described in more detail in Chapter 2, existentialism is an approach to counseling based on strong philosophical roots. An existential therapist believes current maladjusted behavior is a reflection of the patient's unwillingness to
face the issues of human existence, namely death, responsibility,
loneliness, and meaninglessness. Responsibility assumption is
seen as the key to any change and the stress in existential therapy
is on the present. It tends to be a highly confrontational approach with the therapist pointing out and encouraging the living of life as it is and not what the client would like it to be.

3. *Rational therapy.* Developed by Ellis (1975), rational therapy
places heavy emphasis on the cognitive. How we feel is dependent on how we think. It is not the event that is important but
how we interpret the event. It is assumed that the client has the
ability to look rationally at his irrational behavior, and the client-
therapist relationship is not considered an important feature of
this approach. The therapist uses a great deal of confrontation
and persuasion to convince the client of his irrational ideas underlying the self-defeating behavior.

4. *Behavioral counseling.* In behavioral counseling the client's behavior is seen as a set of conditioned responses and the counselor
is seen as a conditioning agent. A goal is agreed on by both the
clinician and the client; the therapist then lays out a program

that involves a series of successive approximations to the desired behavior. Each approximation is reinforced by a suitable reward. The relationship between counselor and client is not paramount to the success of this approach. The counselor is seen as an advisor helping set up a counterconditioning program.

5. *Person-centered counseling.* Developed and articulated most forcefully by Rogers within the humanistic frame of reference, person-centered counseling maintains that maladjusted behavior is caused by the person not having learned—because of poor teaching and parenting—to trust the self-actualizing drive that is within each of us. The vehicle of change is the relationship established with the therapist, which is characterized by warmth, acceptance, and congruence. Rogers (1961) has written of the three conditions necessary for growth: that the counselor be congruent, that he develop an unconditional positive regard for the client, and that he listen empathetically. (The last skill involves reflecting rather than intepreting what the person is saying.) The humanness of the counselor is very much at issue, and counselor responsibility is limited to establishing the facilitative relationship.

These are very briefly the five general approaches to counseling. To contrast them, we can use an example of a person going to a counselor with the desire to give up smoking. If he went to a psychoanalyst, the therapist might be very interested in the patient's early sucking behavior and could possibly see smoking as a reflection of an anal-oral conflict. An existential therapist might see the smoking as a responsibility-assumption issue and would then confront the person on his choosing to smoke. A rational therapist would draw up lists of the reasons for smoking and the arguments against smoking, and would discuss the lists with the patient. A behavioral therapist would devise a plan of cigarette reduction and periodic rewards for meeting the reduction criteria. A person-centered therapist might begin by asking the client what he feels needs to be done for him to give up smoking.

I have heard student clinicians being told by a supervisor that when in doubt they should counsel in a nondirective, person-centered manner, the assumption being that this method will do the least harm. I think this advice is bad because the nondirective approach generates a great deal of anger as it violates client expectation. The "safest" approach by far, I think, is the cognitive approach. People go to a counselor expecting advice; therefore, even if it is bad advice, they have, unfortunately, been getting and surviving from bad advice most of their lives.

No experimental evidence supports the superiority of any one of these approaches. The variables that need to be controlled in order to determine scientifically which is a better approach (e.g., counselor competency, purity of counselor theory, level of client maladjustment, and degree of and measurement of change) are so immense as currently to preclude any meaningful research into therapeutic efficacy. We are reduced to selecting a particular approach because it is most congenial to our personality and to our world view. The client behavior exists, and it is a matter of which therapeutic lens the counselor selects in order to see it. The counselor can also select different lenses at different times: that is, he can be quite eclectic.

COUNSELING AND THE FIELD OF COMMUNICATION DISORDERS

The speech pathologist/audiologist cannot divorce himself from the process of counseling. The most significant resource that a counselor brings to the helping relationship is himself. The importance of the congruent professional far exceeds the value of any diagnostic test or specific techniques in counseling. If the literature on the desirable personality characteristics of the counselor were examined, it would appear that no one would qualify unless one could also qualify for sainthood. It is not necessary to be an entirely self-actualized person to be an effective counselor. I think one needs to have a deep interest in people and a sensitivity to others. One needs to be a caring individual who does not impose his beliefs on others, who maintains a constant awareness of self, and who does not hide behind the artificiality of being a professional.

At workshops I am frequently asked in one form or another, "Can counseling by a speech pathologist damage the client?" I think this question reflects the underlying fear caused by the inadequate training in counseling received by speech-language pathologists and audiologists. Webster (1966) addressed the problem quite well when she wrote about counseling parents.

If counseling means the imposition of prescriptions without care for the person for whom they are prescribed one may indeed do damage. The non-accepting, non-compassionate clinician runs the risk of hurting parents; so does the one who focuses concern on the child to the exclusion of concern for the parents. The speech pathologist or audiologist who leaves to others the interpretation of the information his field has to offer may do parents great harm. The same can be said for the clinician with limited knowledge who gives faulty information.

On the other hand, it is virtually impossible for one person to damage another by listening to him, by trying to understand what the world looks like to him, by permitting him to express what is in him and by honestly giving him the information he needs. In this view of counseling, the clinician serves as an accepting listener. He delays his judgment and tries to accept parents as they are and as they will become (p. 337).

COUNSELING TECHNIQUE

Good counseling technique flows from personality; it is seamless. Technique should not be readily apparent to the person being counseled nor to an observer. This is not to say that there is no technique or that there is no discipline to be learned by the student. As the counselor gains more experience and becomes more secure, technique is incorporated into personality; the skill then becomes unconscious. I find that I frequently have to invent a reason why I did something when a student observer asks me in postevaluation sessions. If I am conscious of technique, I become mechanical and the technique fails because it interferes with the authenticity of the relationship. Counseling is not a mantle that the professional puts on when a client is present and then discards for the rest of his life; it is an attitude, something that is lived. I do not see how one can be a caring, responsive person only within the context of a client-professional relationship.

Technique should not be bound to a particular philosophy. Although I like to think of myself as a humanist I find I use techniques that fit well within behavioral or rational-emotive therapy. I think one does not do something because of identification with a particular therapy, but rather because the evidence based on clinical experience has tended to indicate that this is the way to be most helpful to the other person. Arbuckle (1970) has the following thoughts on this subject:

Thus, in the long run, it would seem that the effective counselor is one who has worked out for himself, through the experience of experimentation, the means by which he can most effectively use himself in a human interaction known as counseling. His orientation has been eclectic, rather than parochial and while his own life is in a constant state of movement and change, he has learned that there are certain modes of operation which are most effective for him, thus there is a degree of consistency in his operation as a counselor. While he is open to consider any means that will work with the client he is aware that his own limitations are such that he cannot be all things for all people. He is acceptant of the thought that there is no model, no method, no technique, which will be consistently successful for him with any other human individual who may come to him as a client (p. 291).

COUNSELOR CONTROL VIA RESPONSE

In a counseling relationship I wait to see what issues are on the client's mind before making a clinical judgment as how best to proceed. There are no stupid questions, only ill-judged responses. The nondirective or person-centered approach affords a great deal of counselor control. The way in which the counselor elects to respond will to a large extent determine the future course of that interaction. The timing of a response is critical. There are times when a client can make good use of content and there are other times when it is very inappropriate. A father of a deaf child might ask "Are there no adequate services for deaf children in this state?" I might respond to this statement by

1. Telling him about the services that are available and offering him a directory of services (content response).
2. Asking him how he came to have that opinion (counterquestion).
3. Commenting, "That must frighten you when you think about services for your child" (affect response).
4. Telling him "no" and then commenting on what a wonderful opportunity this presents for him to get involved in establishing suitable programs (perceptual alteration response).
5. Telling him about my experience trying to find services for my child (sharing self).
6. Responding with a clinical "uh huh" (affirmation).

None of these responses is necessarily the "best" one. (I have delineated six possible responses, which seem to me to be the most clinically facilitative, although the actual number of possible responses is probably infinite.) Each response is appropriate within the context of the relationship. Each response will move the relationship into a different dimension, and appropriateness is determined by a clinical judgment of the therapeutic context. The timing of the response is critical as are the many nonverbal features—tone of voice, facial expression, and body language. Let us look at each response in a bit more detail.

Content Response. The content response is the most common and generally keeps the relationship at an expected and rather predictable level. In the initial stages of a relationship, it is important for the establishment of credibility; in the latter stages it is necessary for the making of appropriate decisions. Generally content relationships are short-term. When the professional has a limited amount of time, content will predominate and tend to keep waiting rooms clear. A professional has the responsibility to keep current regarding his information and to identify fact from opinion—not an easy task. Content has immense value when it is used appropriately.

Counterquestion. I have found that people seldom want advice. What they are usually seeking is confirmation of a position or a decision that they have already made. Instead of revealing that decision they often ask a question, and hope that I will confirm their position. The safest response to a confirmation question is to ask a question in turn. The counterquestion thus will force the person to reveal his position. If one treats a confirmation question as a content question then one is very likely to put one's foot in one's mouth. For example, in one of my programs a Spanish-speaking mother of a deaf child asked me if she had to speak

English at home. I resisted the temptation to tell her that it would be less confusing for her child if she did (she could figure that out for herself) and instead responded by asking her what she wanted to do. The woman responded that if we made her speak English at home she would not come. I told her our policy was to speak English in the nursery and that she would have to decide what she wanted to do at home. One month later she decided to speak English at home.

It was a relief to me to realize that I did not have to answer questions (I think this was a holdover from my school days when I was rewarded by answering my teacher's questions and thus I could prove how smart I was).

Confirmation questions also are used to forestall rejection. A question is a low-risk contribution to an interaction: the questioner does not have to reveal himself, instead he is asking the other person to make a revelation. For example, when I am asked if I am busy tonight I usually respond by asking if the questioner had something in mind for me to do. Embedded in almost all questions is a statement, and I need to be sensitive enough to respond to the statement or at least to elicit that statement.

For me, the best indicator of the trust level in a relationship is the number of question-answer interactions. In initial stages of a relationship, where trust is not high, there are usually a great many questions. As the relationship develops and grows the client becomes more willing to offer statements and observations. The professional can facilitate this therapeutic movement by not always answering questions and supplying content. The counterquestion can be a powerful tool for moving the relationship beyond the initial stages.

Affect Response. The affect response appears risky, but actually it is not. It is responding to what Rogers calls "the faint knocking." By listening very carefully and trying to see the world as the client sees it and reflecting the feelings back to him, the counselor can cause the relationship to be opened up—sometimes very dramatically. The appropriate affect response greatly increases the intimacy level in a relationship. I have found that even an inaccurate response is not harmful; it generally forces the person to clarify further his feelings, and in the process of clarification I can generally understand him better.

The affect response is very potent in building a counseling relationship. Caring is conveyed by our willingness to listen and be responsive to what the person says and also to what the person cannot quite bring himself to say. Rogers calls this empathetic listening and it would appear to be a readily teachable technique. Unfortunately, empathetic listening is often abused and can come across as parroting and mechanical in the hands of someone who has learned the form but not the substance of the humanistic approach.

The affect response requires considerable follow-up; it is not usually a response that one gives when there is limited time. I find responding at the affect level is usually more appropriate in the initial stages of contact and diagnosis. It allows for a ventilation of the feelings and for the alleviation of some of the secondary feelings that accompany the strong affect surrounding a catastrophic illness. The wife, for example, who feels very angry at her husband for having a stroke, can be given the opportunity to talk about her feelings of anger without feeling guilty. In later stages, when affect is not so predominant, I generally give more content responses or perceptual alteration responses.

Perceptual Alteration Response. The timing of the perceptual alteration response has to be fairly precise and it cannot be used too frequently or you will be accused of being a "Pollyanna." It is immensely effective in mobilizing action by getting the person to look at the positive side. So much of our orientation is to the problem that we seldom see the challenge that is present in the situation. The perceptual alteration response encourages responsibility assumption. The parent in the group who complains about the "dumb questions" he gets from strangers who see his child's hearing aids can be brought up short by the response "What a marvelous opportunity to educate someone about deafness."

Professionals can also benefit from the perceptual alteration response when analyzing their client relationships. For example, behavior can be interpreted as stubborn or as determined—stubbornness is the negative side of determination. If the clinician is always looking at the stubborn side he will have a negative view of the client. A determined client has a much greater chance of success than a stubborn client.

I think that we seldom consider or call attention to client strengths, so often are we looking at their deficits. Very often it helps, when I supervise student clinicians, to ask them "What does this child have going for him?" and then "How can we capitalize on those strengths?" When we focus on the client's strengths, somehow the problem begins to disappear far faster than when we emphasize his deficits.

Sharing Self. It is very valuable for the client to realize that the professional is also a person who has concerns, fears, and a life outside of the clinic. It helps the client assume responsibility and prevents the professional from being elevated to the guru category. The timing of this response is also critical: if it is done too early the professional can lose credibility at a time when credibility establishment is critical for the relationship. This response can also be taken as a prescription by the client rather than as a sharing response. The professional must make clear that this is how he is dealing with a particular issue and it in no way implies that the client should do likewise. It is very hard to do this in initial interactions unless the client has a strong inner locus of control and is able to evaluate the input.

Affirmation Response. I am reminded of the countless cartoons featuring a psychoanalyst: a patient is on the couch doing the talking and the psychiatrist is asleep. Presumably progress is being made. Very often the client just needs a sounding board; he needs permission to talk and to experience his feelings without judgment. The "uh huh" response with appropriate nonverbal behavior can be very helpful in unleashing the client's feelings. The "uh huh" is also an affirmation that the counselor has heard the client and is an invitation for the client to continue. I have a poster in my office given to me by a group of students which says, "It often shows a fine command of language to say nothing." Sometimes the most facilitative remarks are the ones that you do not deliver.

The clinician has a wide array of potential responses; which one he selects will determine the direction of the relationship. There are no "right" responses, only different roads to travel. If the response you give moves the relationship in a fruitful direction, then it is appropriate. It is also quite possible to recover from taking a less fruitful route. I have found that if something is important it keeps coming up, and a feeling is seldom lost—it just gets reworked and emerges again.

COUNSELOR FEEDBACK

How the counselor feels about the client is a valuable source of data, which the counselor should judiciously share with the client. Although this sharing can be very facilitative for client growth, it must always be done within a context of support and the timing must also be precise. For example, in a student clinician group, one participant was especially verbose; she continually repeated herself. Toward the end of one of her monologues, I interrupted and commented: "———, I find your initial statements and thoughts very interesting, and then when you keep repeating yourself I find myself getting bored and emotionally distanced from you." The comment allowed her to begin talking about how other people had given her this feedback and that her verbosity reflected her loneliness and her insecurity. The rest of the group, which up to that point was sitting there with glazed-over eyes, began to give her more feedback and the group then moved into a fruitful discussion of loneliness and the things they sometimes do that distance other people.

When feedback is given, it is very important that the person who delivers the feedback comment about his own feelings. Thus, I did not say "You talk too much," which would have put her on the defensive, I spoke only about what was going on in my mind. At that point in time the problem was mine not hers, and as long as I talk about myself I am always an expert.

COGNITIVE RESTRUCTURING

Cognitive restructuring relies heavily on the rational-emotive approach developed by Ellis and Harper (1975). In many ways Ellis pioneered the use of general semantics in psychotherapy. This approach pays very careful attention to the language that a person is using and examines the underlying irrational assumptions of those linguistic constructs. The major irrational ideas that underlie rational-emotive therapy are

1. It is a dire necessity for an adult human being to be loved or approved of by virtually every "significant other" in his community.
2. A person should be thoroughly competent, adequate, and achieving in all possible respects if he is to consider himself worthwhile, and he is utterly worthless if he is incompetent in any way.
3. Certain people can be labeled bad, wicked, or villainous, and they deserve severe blame or punishment for their sins.
4. It is awful or catastrophic when things are not the way an individual would very much like them to be.
5. Human unhappiness is externally caused and individuals have little or no ability to control their sorrows and disturbances.
6. If something is or may be dangerous or fearsome, one should be terribly concerned about it and should keep dwelling on the possibility of its occurrence.
7. It is easier to avoid certain life difficulties and self-responsibilities than it is to face them.
8. An individual should be dependent on others and needs someone stronger than himself on whom to rely.
9. A person's past history is an all-important determinant of his present behavior, and because something once strongly affected his life, it should continue to do so.
10. An individual should become quite upset over other people's problems and disturbances.
11. There is invariably a correct, precise, and perfect solution to human problems, and it is catastrophic if this perfect solution is not found.

I find these irrational ideas occurring in almost all of my professional contacts and they seem to be a major source of unhappiness. These irrational ideas are reflected in the language people use to describe their problems, for example, the use of the word *can't* when it is really a "choose not to" situation, as in "I can't tell my pediatrician how angry I am" or "I can't use my new speech on the telephone." Other language changes that I find valuable are:

Should and *ought* changed to *want to* or *not want to*
  as in: "I should use my new voice."
      "I want to (or do not want to) use my new voice."
Have to changed to *want to* or *choose to*
  as in: "I have to stay home and not meet people."
      "I want to stay home" or "I choose to stay home."
We, us, society, and so on, changed to *I*
  as in: "We are unhappy with this class."
      "I am unhappy with this class."
To be verbs modified
  as in: "I am a dumb person."
      "I did a dumb thing and I am still a smart person."
But changed to *and* (as in all the *yes . . . but* sentences)
  as in: "I want to speak in public but I am afraid."
      "I want to speak in public and I am afraid."

All of these linguistic changes force the person to assume responsibility for his behavior or for thinking about that behavior. Underlying rational-emotive therapy, as with all other therapies, is responsibility assumption.

Ellis has a very confrontive, directive style and feels that it is the responsibility of the therapist to convince the patient of his irrational behavior. He is not above giving homework. I find that I can use these ideas in a much less confrontational style, that the linguistic changes can be made gently. The timing is critical. I will seldom make linguistic changes in initial stages or when affect is high; these changes require cognition, and the person very quickly loses the feeling and train of thought. Trust needs to be high because the linguistic alterations can be seen as interfering and annoying if not done with sensitivity.

The irrational ideas that I must be universally liked and that a competent and worthwhile person makes no mistakes I find particularly valuable in working with student clinicians (also professionals). The student clinicians generally try so hard to be liked that they are unwilling to offend their clients in any way. This means that they tend to meet client expectations rather than their own. The fear of making mistakes severely limits personal and professional growth and seems to be almost epidemic in student populations. I think that this is a direct reflection of the poor teaching methods that our students have been subjected to, because almost every professional group that I work with deals with these same issues.

In working with client populations I find that the evasion of responsibility and dependency issues are the most prevalent. I look for evidence of the client seeking to evade responsibility by becoming dependent on me or by avoiding dealing with the issue of the communication disorder and call it to his attention. One of the major ways of alerting him (and me) is by careful attention to his language, which reflects his perception of the world and of our relationship.

SILENCE

Silence is an important component of any therapeutic relationship. A long, embarrassed silence frequently occurs very early in my clinical interactions. Because clients generally expect the professional to direct conversation, when I do not take the lead a silence ensues. It is vital that I do not break this silence. It tells the other person that if he wants something to happen in this relationship, he is going to have to act. The silence is a primary vehicle for promoting responsibility assumption and it is vital that I do not take that responsibility from the client. Terror of this silence initially forces many young clinicians to act; they then become role-bound to make things happen while the client sits back and watches.

Silences are generally uncomfortable in conventional relationships. I can remember the long painful silences I had as an adolescent on blind dates while I thought frantically of something to say. (I suspect the girl was similarly occupied but I was too concerned with my own discomfort to think of hers.) The discomfort generated by the silence can be used by the clinician to motivate action by the client. I am fortified by the knowledge of what I am doing and the value of this technique, and this enables me to outwait most clients. The general reaction of the client to the silence is anger, and if this surfaces it becomes a useful vehicle for discussing role expectations.

Later on in relationships, the silences that occur are of a more reflective nature. They are quite comfortable. As intimacy develops the silences become a very valuable learning time for processing material. Where there is silence there is usually growth. Cook (1964) analyzed the amount of silences in taped therapy sessions and found that the more successful outcomes had more silences than those therapy sessions judged to be less successful. Sometimes talking can be used as a smokescreen to hide feelings and in the silence one is often forced to confront self and to experience feelings.

I like the Montaigne quote, "A bore is someone who takes my solitude and gives me nothing in return." I resent it when my introspection is interrupted by chatter, and I relish the companionship of a thoughtful silence.

CONTRACTING

Contracting is a technique used extensively in the behavioral approach; essentially it is making explicit all of the assumptions underlying the relationship. The client is required to be explicit about what is wanted from the clinician, and the clinician is very explicit about what will be done or what will not be done for the client. Initial sessions of the interaction are devoted almost solely to the contracting issue. Periodically, as the relationship progresses, time is taken to renegotiate the contract if needed.

I find it very important to delineate carefully what I expect from clients. Many relationships fail because of expectations that are implicit and are not complementary. Clients, for example, who expect the therapist to rescue them, and a teacher who expects the parents to be very active will have a difficult time unless they can negotiate the differences. If the issue of expectations is not dealt with, the relationship will deteriorate and anger will develop although it will probably not be directed at its appropriate source.

Basically a contract determines the duration of the relationship, what it will entail, and its purpose. Contracts do not have to be detailed or legalistic, but they have to be understood by everybody. In particular, I think the time issue needs to be very clear. Before I start a session I am always explicit about how much time I have in a given encounter, and I am very rigid about terminating when I have said I would. I will very seldom extend a session beyond the contracted time. The limited amount of time then serves as an impetus (death awareness) to the clients to work toward solving their problem. If I had an open-ended commitment with closure occurring at some unspecified time, clients would tend to avoid dealing with painful material, thinking that they could get to it at some vague future date. It is no accident that more and more affect-laden material is revealed at the session's end than at the beginning.

I am also open to renegotiating contracts. As relationships change, needs change and I have to be cognizant of that. I never unilaterally change a relationship; the change has to be discussed and agreed on. It sometimes comes to pass that neither I nor the client can arrive at a mutually satisfactory contract. When this happens we terminate. I generally will assume the responsibility of referring the client (if he wishes) to someone who I think can meet his needs. I have ceased trying to be all things to all people and I recognize that there are some people I cannot help, or more accurately, choose not to help, because to do so would violate my own personal values. Invariably, this occurs around responsibility assumption, where the client persistently wants me to do much more than I think is prudent for effecting growth.

SOME OTHER CONSIDERATIONS
Clinical Applications of Humanism. The direct clinical application of humanism is not always apparent and is sometimes difficult to apply. A behavioral approach with its highly specified, operationally defined behaviors leaves the clinician with a structure to hold onto and relate to. Progress is known and goals are very clearly specified. A cognitive, content-oriented approach is also relatively easy to grasp and administer. The clinician has the content from his academic experience and can control events within therapy by keeping the relationship and activities in the

cognitive realm. The humanistic approach with its assumption of client strength and client power means that the clinician gives up control of events. It means that the clinician will have to follow the lead of the client and be prepared to meet the needs as they arise in spontaneous interaction, which places a much greater burden on the clinician. It also becomes difficult for me to recommend specific behaviors for the clinician to follow. In one sense the clinician can behave in any way that events dictate as long as he respects and empowers the client. I would like to indicate some things that can be done in both diagnosis and therapy, which will encourage client responsibility assumption and facilitate the counseling and therapeutic process within a humanistic framework.

Diagnosis. I think that it is vital for both the client and the family to participate fully in the diagnostic process. I think it is a big mistake for the clinician to take the client off somewhere and administer diagnostic tests and then return and try to communicate the results to the family. It is often very difficult for the family to grasp the terminology and to emotionally accept what is being said. This kind of diagnostic protocol leaves the way open for the family to practice denial and it severely limits the counseling function. The counseling is immediately placed in a cognitive realm with the clinician having to explain the results.

In my clinical audiology work with a young child, I immediately enlist the parents as codiagnosticians. I start by asking the parents what they think the problem is and at some point tell them that we will decide together as I need their help in determining the hearing status of their child. We then go together into the soundproof room and adjust the testing until we both agree that the child responded or did not respond. At all times I explain how loud the sound is and what the frequency of the sound is.

After the testing is completed I turn to my codiagnosticians and ask what they thought their child could hear. If there is some disagreement between us we return to the room and see if we can reach an agreement.

Once agreement has been reached we can proceed to talk about feelings. If we have decided that the child could not hear I usually ask parents how they are feeling. Typically I get a response such as "numb." At that point I may give parents some help in the affect area by telling them that "some parents have felt at that time like they were hit by a truck." Usually parents at this point have almost no questions and generally they want to go somewhere and cry. I generally give them the address and phone number of a parent of an older deaf child. (They seldom call as the denial mechanism starts working very quickly.) I also schedule another meeting with them as soon as possible. On subsequent meetings more and more affect emerges as the trust builds in our relationship, and more content is exchanged as the parents ask more questions. Parents who have reminisced with me about that first time they were in the soundproof room with me have said how very hard it was to sit there and hear those sounds and not see their child respond. They could no longer deny that their child was deaf. They also felt closer to me as we went through the process together. While it was painful they were also very glad that I was there.

With hard-of-hearing adults and older hearing-impaired children I always credit highly what they are telling me. I never select a hearing aid for them; they choose their own after trying several clinic models. I never try to convince them to wear a hearing aid. All phases of the testing are explained to them and their choices are respected. All accompanying family are part of the whole clinical process and are not left to wait in the waiting room. I think that speech and language diagnostics can be carried out in a similar vein.

Therapy. I have limited therapeutic experience. It would seem to me, however, that in order to apply a humanistic approach to the therapy situation clinicians have to modify the use of the lesson plan. The first session and perhaps each session would begin by asking the client what he would like to work on and how he thought that could be best accomplished. Together the client and the therapist could evolve the lesson plan. Both would have an equal opportunity and right to decide on the therapeutic activities. At all times the clinician should trust the client to know what is best for himself and should allow the client full rein to explore therapeutic possibilities. This is not to say that there are no limits set. The clinician also retains full power and has rights that must be respected. The rules for working together are mutually agreed on.

The client who is not able to communicate, such as a young child or a severely disabled adult, will present the clinician with a major therapeutic challenge. The clinician will need to be very sensitive to the nonverbal behavior. All clients communicate or try to communicate. We need to be able to "read" our clients' behavior (this is also true of clients who can communicate verbally). It is also necessary to recognize that in many cases the family needs to be involved in therapy and the "client" can or should be the normally communicating family member. (This concept will be discussed in greater detail in Chaps. 6 and 7.)

Effectiveness of Counseling. A frequent mistake made by the neophyte counselor is in thinking that the goal of counseling is to eliminate pain—to make people who are in pain feel better. This idea is very natural and desirable in a helping professional; however, it is not healthy to be responsible for another's pain, and by trying to make the person feel better the clinician often invalidates the client. It is seldom useful to tell or imply that a person should not feel that way. This strategy generally only helps people to feel guilty about their emotional pain.

The emotional pain is normal. I expect people to feel sad when bad things happen to them; if I do not encounter pain in people who have a communication disorder and their families, I wonder how they are dealing with this catastrophe. A mother of a newly diagnosed deaf child told me that she was "doing this badly." By this she meant that she was crying several hours every day. I assured her that she was not doing badly, she was reacting normally. Professionals can be most helpful to their clients by taking away the negative feelings about the pain that they are experiencing; however, we cannot take away the pain. A core of pain will remain in any permanent disability.

The goal of counseling then is to detach the feelings from self-defeating behavior. I never judge feelings; they just exist and I accept them. We can, however, work together on what constitutes constructive behavior. Thus a parent who says "I can feel guilty *and* I can still act in a way that is in my own and my child's best interest" has grown successfully. Clients find, over time and with careful professional attention, that feelings no longer control them, and "guilty" parents do not have to overprotect their child. Client behavior has to be the ultimate criterion by which we judge the effectiveness of counseling.

Professional Humility. If one is to counsel from a humanistic frame of reference, which is accepting and not prescribing, then one must learn a professional humility. Fortunately, for me it occurred rather early in my counseling career.

Johnny was a 2-year-old hearing-impaired child in one of our first nursery groups. He would enter the nursery with his thumb in his mouth and his little finger stuck up one nostril. The finger stayed in his nostril the whole 2 hours of the nursery day, which included 30 minutes of individual speech therapy. As it is rather hard to relate to someone with his thumb in his mouth and almost impossible for the child to speak, Johnny never participated in nursery activities, preferring to watch the other children. The staff became convinced that he was an emotionally disturbed child. One goal of therapy was to condition Johnny to remove his thumb from his mouth; another goal was to get Johnny's parents to seek psychiatric help. I assumed the latter responsibility and would sit next to his mother during nursery and during speech therapy pointing out to her how deficient Johnny was compared with the other children.

The mother refused to see any of the nonparticipatory behavior as abnormal. She always seemed to have an explanation for his behavior. Consequently, we were unsuccessful on both counts: the thumb remained in the child's mouth until the end of the semester and the parents decided, much to our dismay and over our objections, to put Johnny in a hearing nursery school and provide him with individual speech and language therapy. So with much staff head-shaking the parents left the program. Several months later, I chanced to meet the father socially and of course wanted to know how Johnny was doing. He told me with a big smile on his face, "Johnny has kissed his teacher." Well, I thought, at least they got his hand out of his mouth—or did they? The family moved to the West Coast and, as often happens in this business, we lost all contact.

Several years later I happened to be at a meeting on the West Coast and met Johnny's mother. (She had decided to become a speech pathologist.) I found out that Johnny was attending his neighborhood school, fully mainstreamed, and—as shown by his recent achievement test—was operating at grade level. His mother brought his latest report card, which indicated very normal social skills. Fortunately, this family had enough strength to resist my manipulation. I often think of this case and wonder how many of my early prognostications were so far off the mark. I suspect a great many. The professional does not have access to all the relevant data. The parent or client knows much more of the really important data to make life decisions, and I have learned, although at times it has been painful to my professional ego, to trust people to make their own decisions. I figure that they know what is best for themselves.

Humility helps the counselor develop listening skills. Once the counselor recognizes his own limitations, he can put aside his own point of view about what the person should do. If the counselor has a point of view, he then stops listening fully; he will listen only for the weakness so as to present his arguments and thus have his point of view prevail. I did not hear Johnny's mother. I thought only that this was a mother who was denying that she had a multiply handicapped child, and I filtered everything she said through that perception. I did not respond to her concerns or fears or credit her content; instead we were engaged in an adversarial relationship, which did not grow and, more importantly, which did not benefit her child.

Counselor Mistakes. I have made mistakes on many occasions. Usually these errors are not so much failures of commission as failures to capitalize on a very cogent situation. I almost always recover from my insensitivities and gaffes. I bring them up at the next session or, if I am really bothered by them, I call up the client and apologize. These apologies have helped relationships because they convey my humanity and my vulnerability, both of which contribute to client growth.

The failure to capitalize on situations, however, is a reflection on my lack of skill at the time. I cannot guarantee to clients that I will always be skillful. I can only promise that I will be doing the best I know how to do and will continue to be a learning and growing professional. My errors are personal "nuggets of gold" (although they may not be seen that way by clients), because they show me what I still need to learn.

I have observers in all my parent groups and after each session, we have a postmortem with an eye to what I might have done differently. I find these sessions very helpful, and many times I can recover a mistake, although it is never quite the same as having acted at that particular time. These are the "should have dones" that I think all professionals carry with them. Early in my career I tape-recorded sessions and listened carefully to the playbacks, which helped me to identify areas that I needed to work on. In more than 20 years of doing this, I still find areas that I need to work on. They keep me going and I always feel professionally challenged.

The Unattractive Client. Occasionally I find a client toward whom it is difficult for me to develop an unconditional positive regard. These clients are like weeds in the garden and bring to mind the Emerson quote: "A weed is a plant whose virtues have not yet been discovered." I have to keep searching with these "weeds" to find those virtues. I have found that with care and patience some of my ugliest weeds have turned into beautiful flowers; some unfortunately have remained weeds.

B I B L I O G R A P H Y

Arbuckle, D. *Counseling: Philosophy, Theory and Practice* (2nd ed.). Boston: Allyn & Bacon, 1970.

Cook, J. Silences in psychotherapy. *J. Counseling Psychol.* 11:42, 1964.

Ellis, A., and Harper, R. *A New Guide to Rational Living*. Englewood Cliffs, N.J.: Prentice-Hall, 1975.

Rogers, C. *On Becoming a Person*. Boston: Houghton Mifflin, 1961.

Webster, E. Parent counseling by speech pathologists and audiologists. *J. Speech Hear. Disord.* 31:331, 1966.

CHAPTER 5

GROUPS

I have a very strong bias in favor of groups, which I would like to share at the outset of this chapter. I feel that groups are a very efficacious means of counseling. In fact I seldom do individual counseling as I find it less effective. Within an individual session I have to be very wise and very alert—there is no help. Within the group setting many resources are available and I do not have to be so all-encompassing; invariably when I am at a loss someone within the group rescues me. I think that within a group there is marvelous health, strength, and a collective wisdom, which supersedes the wisdom of any one member. The task of the leader is to unleash that wisdom.

Although my group work has been mainly with parents of hearing-impaired children, I have had some experience with parents of children with other handicaps and I have worked with groups of hard-of-hearing adults. I have also led student-clinician groups and groups of practicing speech-language pathologists and audiologists.

GROUPS IN SPEECH PATHOLOGY AND AUDIOLOGY

It is difficult to determine from reading the literature on communication disorders just how extensively groups are used. I suspect they are used much more frequently than the literature would indicate. There appear to be two types of groups: a therapy group and a counseling group. The therapy group composed of speech-language-defective individuals is used fairly frequently and has a long history. This group is convened to work on a specific speech or language problem. Backus and Beasley (1951), writing more than 30 years ago, found group therapy of speech-defective children gave superior results as compared to individual therapy. Recently Albertini and colleagues (1983) found that deaf adolescents did as well working on their speech within a group as did a control group who had individual therapy. In the years between these two reports, many others were published that supported the notion of group therapy if for no other reason than better utilization of therapist time. I suspect that many therapy groups are started and maintained in the hope of reducing the therapist's waiting list.

Of concern here is the counseling group (this is not to say that counseling is not part of a therapy group), which may or may not be composed of speech-language-defective individuals. This group has an implicit mandate to deal with feelings. Many counseling groups in practice, I suspect, stay with content because of the therapist's insecurity. The groups are convened and conceived as places where individuals can talk about the feelings generated by having a speech-language defect or having a relative who has a speech-language defect. Webster (1968, 1977) has written extensively about counseling parents of speech-defective children within a group context. Dee (1981) uses a group context to counsel parents of deaf children. Bardach (1969) found groups very helpful with spouses of aphasic patients. Emerson (1980) found positive changes in the self-esteem of the spouses of patients with aphasia as a result of group counseling, while Singler (1982) found that groups can be very helpful for the stroke patients themselves. Schein (1982) reported on counseling groups for deaf adults. Apparently these groups are used quite frequently with varying degrees of success depending on how well the group can overcome the communication problem.

Outside of the field of communication disorders, groups are used extensively. Seligman (1982), reporting on counseling special populations within a group format, describes groups of special populations, which have included cancer patients, the physically disabled, the elderly, drug abusers, prison populations, the mentally retarded, the visually impaired, and alcoholics. Probably the most extensive use of group techniques has been in the field of psychotherapy. The definitive text to date in group psychotherapy has been written by Yalom (1975). In this text Yalom identified 11 interdependent curative factors in group therapy. I think that eight of these factors have wide applicability in counseling groups within the communication disorders field. (The three other curative factors that Yalom lists—the development of socialization techniques, imitative behavior, and the corrective recapitulization of the primary family group—I think are either contained within previous factors or are more appropriate for psychotherapeutic groups.)

CURATIVE FACTORS IN GROUPS
Instillation of Hope. By seeing how others have improved, the client can come to feel that there is hope for her. To see how oth-

ers have overcome their adversity buoys up others. There is always someone in a group who is "up" and lifts the spirits of the others. In fact, faith and hope may be the only curative factors one needs: witness the efficacy of faith healers and placebo therapy. There is also the faith that the therapist has in the group process itself, which is transmitted to the clients. I personally have an almost mystical belief in the power of the group for healing and growth.

Universality. The group helps the person recognize that she is not alone in her feelings and perceptions. More often than not, parents of a disabled child feel that they are crazy or sick for feeling a particular way (which usually involves wishing the child were dead) and when they find out that other parents have felt the same way, they feel relief: they are not alone, and they are not crazy. Universality is a feeling that you can only get within a group format and is very much a factor in dealing with the existential issue of loneliness.

Imparting of Information. The information is provided not only by the leader, although many groups are structured so that the leader provides most of the content, but also by the other members of the group. I am always astonished at how much clients already know and sometimes some of the least articulate members in the group come up with marvelous, unique solutions. I am also struck by how rarely advice-giving is directly beneficial to a group member, although it is frequently offered within the group. Of much more lasting value is the sharing of experiences and the consequent knowledge gained. Advice-giving, I think, is indirectly seen as conveying a mutual interest and a caring and as such serves a vital function in the group. All groups, however, should and almost always do leave the participants more informed than when the group started. There is a collective wisdom within a group that is greater than the knowledge of any one participant.

Altruism. Very much related to the imparting of information is that the participants in the group get a chance to help one another. Because we are dealing with the disabled, we find that they rarely have the chance to help anyone, which diminishes self-esteem. Being a helper enables one to receive help without a concomitant loss of self-esteem. Within the group the members are immensely helpful to one another. They offer support, reassurance, and insights. I find, for example, that parents of disabled children will listen much more attentively to another parent than they do to me. Another parent has a different credibility that I can never duplicate. A frequent end result of a successful counseling group is the desire—and the translation of that desire into action—to help similarly disabled populations. This is a healthy result, which moves the group away from an almost morbid self-absorption and allows the individuals to grow.

Interpersonal Learning. Humans have always lived in groups; in fact, our survival depends on our ability to live in groups. Yet I find that many of the people I come in contact with (parents of disabled children, student clinicians, speech-language pathologists, audiologists) have poor interpersonal skills, in part, I think, because of poor early learning in their family of origin; that is, they have difficulty communicating with others, being trusting and honest with others, and learning to love more fully. None of this is pathological in the sense that these people are nonfunctional. It is a matter of their being able to get more joy and more satisfaction out of all of their interpersonal interactions. The group can be a very safe vehicle for the participants to enhance their interpersonal learning. They can learn (or more appropriately, relearn) how to be more open and accepting of others and can then take this knowledge from the group context into their other relationships.

Group Cohesiveness. Cohesiveness, a basic property of groups, is very difficult to define and to grasp, yet I think it is an integral factor in successful counseling. It is analogous to the relationship in individual therapy. Cohesiveness is not a curative factor per se, but rather a precondition. Cohesiveness is related to the attractiveness of the group to its members. I know the group will be successful when I can hardly wait for the sessions to start and I look forward to seeing the other members of the group. Cohesiveness is intricately tied to trust: where trust develops, much as in individual therapy, groups come together and growth can occur. Whenever someone in a group reveals a deep secret, which is accepted and amplified by other members of the group, there is a quantum leap in group cohesiveness.

Another intangible factor, an interpersonal attraction that occurs or does not occur in some groups, also determines cohesiveness. Some groups seem to come together very easily and I do not have to work for cohesivness. The members of the group are attracted to one another because of value similarities and, I suspect, some transferences that they bring to the experience. The "chemistry" of the group seems right; it is a good mix of talkers and listeners, and individuals like each other. In other groups cohesiveness is hard to come by—members do not especially like each other or share much with each other. I tend to want to blame the lack of cohesiveness on bad group chemistry and not on my lack of skill. When pressed to the wall, however, I do think that it is a skill issue: I need to pay more careful attention to building trust and cohesiveness in the early stages of the group and to quickly identify when a group is not developing cohesiveness.

Although I think individuals can and do learn even when a group is not cohesive, I think that the learning is greater and much deeper in a cohesive group. Many life-long and close friendships have come about as the result of my being in a group that had a high degree of cohesiveness.

Catharsis. Catharsis, which is closely related to universality, is the expression of the considerable affect that surrounds communication disorders. Almost all participants bring to the group pent-up and stifled feelings, which they have no safe place to express. The group can provide that vehicle for the release and sharing of these feelings. Families of stroke victims, for example, invariably come to feel that they can talk in the group because they can be understood. Professional groups tend to bring their feelings of inadequacy to the fore, and there is a great deal of relief in being able to express these feelings and to be heard and understood by the other members of the group.

Catharsis per se is not a curative factor since just expressing a feeling is not sufficient to promote growth. It is, however, a preliminary to being able to unhook the feelings from the unhealthy behavior. A parent in a group once remarked, "I still feel those feelings but they no longer control me."

Existential Issues. Existential issues are described in detail in Chapter 2. Groups give the individual a chance to work through their death-life enhancement, responsibility assumption–dependency, loneliness-love, and meaningless-commitment issues. Almost all of the personal growth issues that emerge in the groups I lead can be classified under these existential issues. They are a powerful way of looking at individuals and judging personal growth. When groups, and the individuals within groups, are willing to face the existential issues, then growth and change begin.

GROUP GOALS IN COMMUNICATION DISORDERS
All 11 factors can be grouped under three broad categories, which would relate to groups within the field of communication disorders. These group purposes are conveying content, sharing of affect, and personal growth. The goals are contained within the curative factors and need only be discussed briefly here as they relate to communication disorders.

Content. All groups to a certain extent have a content mandate; that is, the convening of the group makes possible the sharing of information and experiences of the members. Learning is unavoidable within a group context, although sometimes what is learned is neither what you expected nor what the leader intended. Groups, I think, proceed best when the leader is not perceived as the sole source of content. This may violate expectations of the group members, but in the long run I think that more is learned from the group when there is a collective responsibility to teach one another. Unfortunately, many groups within the field of communication disorders seem to have content dissemination as their sole purpose and usually this is content supplied by the professional. They are missing much.

Affect Release. Being the parent of a disabled child, having an important family member undergo a catastrophic illness, or having a communication defect will engender a great many feelings that usually have no healthy way of being expressed. Frequently the feelings are repressed—especially anger—which results in depression, or are displaced to others, which impairs interpersonal relationships. The group can become the vehicle for releasing the affect in a safe environment among people who understand those feelings. The group, more than any other vehicle I know, can give sanction and permission to its members to feel their feelings.

Personal Growth. Personal growth is not ordinarily thought of as a responsibility within the discipline of communication disorders, yet I feel that we must address this issue in order to be more effective as professionals. We need to help, for example, parents of disabled children to become more assertive and less compliant when participating with professionals in making educational plans for their child. In order for this to happen the parents (as well as all people with communication disorders) need to have higher self-esteem and a more internal locus of control. People with a communication disorder have to learn to take responsibility for their disability in order to minimize its negative effects on their personal lives. They may learn ways of utilizing their disorder to help others as when they form self-help groups and political action groups to further benefit the handicapped in our society.

The group can be a powerful personal growth vehicle. It can allow individuals to help others, and if the leader is willing to "sit on her wisdom" the group members can take control and therefore learn responsibility assumption. This cannot help but carry over into their everyday lives.

PRINCIPLES OF GROUP FUNCTIONING

Leadership. The leadership of the group becomes a vital factor in determining the success of the group. Groups are an entity unto themselves; that is, each group has its own unique personality and no two groups are ever the same. The principles underlying successful indivivdual counseling are equally applicable to counseling within a group setting. The counselor, from a humanistic point of view, must treat the group with acceptance, genuineness, empathy, and concern. He must be seen as a caring person.

Lieberman and colleagues (1973), in their exhaustive study of encounter groups,* found there were four leadership functions that were directly related to the outcomes.

1. *Emotional stimulation:* accomplished by confronting, modeling, risk-taking, and disclosing self
2. *Caring:* accomplished by offering support, affection, warmth, concern, and genuineness
3. *Meaning attribution:* accomplished by exploring, clarifying, interpreting, and providing a cognitive framework for change
4. *Executive function:* accomplished by setting limits and rules, managing time, and suggesting procedures

The authors found that those leaders who were very high in caring and meaning attribution and who were moderate in emotional stimulation and in executive function were the most successful leaders. Their successes were independent of their theoretical orientation. Groups grew with leaders who cared about them and could give them a cognitive framework for understanding their behavior. Groups were limited in their growth by leaders who were too high or too low on provoking feelings and were too high or too low on executive function. Too little executive function tended to create confused groups while too much executive function tended to create passive groups. Too lit-

Encounter was a term coined by Rogers for those groups that stressed personal growth through the authentic encounter between members. All members of these groups were considered normal and were trying to learn how to get more from their personal relationships. Encounter group is used synonymously with T-group and sensitivity group.

tle emotional stimulation led to devitalized groups, while emotionally overcharged groups were chaotic.

In my experience with parent groups in particular, I have found that it is seldom necessary to provide emotional stimulation. The affect is so high to begin with that, by providing the safe, caring atmosphere, the feelings emerge without any need to provoke the affect.

Establishment of Group Norms. The single most important function of the leader is to set norms for the group. These are the implicit and sometimes very explicit rules by which the group is to function. A group's norms are established very early in the life of the group, and very hard to change once established. The leader establishes the norms by modeling and, especially procedural norms, by stating them explicitly. The most frequently used mechanism for establishing norms in the group is through the reinforcement paradigm. The leader, by virtue of the power accorded to her by the members of the group, uses social approval as a powerful reinforcement agent to ensure group norms. Thus, those behaviors or remarks that she chooses to acknowledge tend to become valued by the group and those behaviors that are not acknowledged tend to be devalued. Most leaders reinforce norms unwittingly based on some deep-seated and unconscious prejudices that they have.

I think the greatest source of failure for me with groups has been in allowing unhealthy group norms to develop and in not acting soon enough to prevent a poor norm from taking hold. For example, in one group that I was leading I was called away to answer the phone (something I do not now allow to happen), and when I returned the parents were having a passionate discussion on which was the best diaper to use on their children. I listened for a while and then very stupidly confronted the group as to why they were wasting their time here discussing such a trivial topic when they could do that elsewhere. The group thereafter became a very low-risk, low-contributing group, one of the dullest groups I had ever worked with. When I was finally able to see what was happening (2 months later—I am a bit slow) I realized that I had established a norm of leader-generated topics. There apparently were, as far as the group was concerned, only certain topics that were appropriate to talk about within the meeting and they had to guess what was acceptable because if they did not they would incur my wrath. The best strategy for them to adopt was to play safe and not risk a new topic. The topics groups select to talk about are never irrelevant; leaders sometimes are.

This group never recovered. If I had it to do over again (a lament most professionals share) I would say, "It must be so hard for you when you have so many choices." This remark might have moved the group to look at all the choices they had to make regarding their children. At the very least I would have done better to have kept quiet and allowed some other members to point out how they were wasting time. In either case, I do not think that I would have had a dull group.

Let us examine some healthy group norms.

Interactional Norm. If the members are to relate and learn from one another, then they have to interact among themselves. Most groups begin with a question directed toward the leader. If she answers the question, another question-and-answer exchange is usually encouraged. This means that the leader can get quickly trapped into providing content via answering the questions and speaking about 50 percent of the time. If the group is to function as a group, the leader has to quickly get away from answering questions and encourage interactions among all the group members. For me, I feel if I take no more than 10 percent of the time it is usually a successful group. The interactional norm allows for the sharing of information and for the helping that can occur among members.

Initiative Norm. I personally think the initiative norm is vital for growth. The group members must learn that if they want something to happen they must make it happen. I come into the group without an agenda and without any topic. What is to be discussed will be determined by the group for that day, and if they wish to sit there and be passive then nothing will happen. Early in the history of a group a silence descends while the group waits to be told what to do and how to proceed. If the leader takes control at this juncture, she begins to establish a norm of a leader-controlled group with the leader taking the initiative. Once this norm is established the members become spectators and the leader begins to feel as if she is doing all the work (she is) and can become very resentful. It is very hard for a professional not to take initiative because it conforms to the implicit expectations of both the professional and the client. I almost never use structured experiences (see p. 130) early in the life of a group because it establishes a leader-initiated group.

Self-Disclosure. Self-disclosure is a necessary component of growth. It is hard for me to see how the participants can learn if they are unwilling to share themselves. I must establish a norm where it is never dangerous to reveal self. When individuals do reveal, they are never penalized and are always supported. Self-disclosure must always be safe, especially when participants, for example, finally reveal their guilty secret. A group will become very cohesive when another parent can say "I always felt that way," or when the other members will accept the secret without saying or implying that the group member should not feel that way. When there are many "should nots" floating around, groups become very inhibited and little self-disclosure occurs thereafter.

In one group I facilitated, a laryngectomized man revealed for the first time that he never used his artificial larynx when he went outside because it embarrassed him. None of the other group members told him that he "should" use his larynx. Instead they listened and expressed to him their understanding of how hard it was to appear so deviant. After a while he began crying and received a great deal of emotional support from the group. Several sessions later he announced to the group that he was now using the larynx in public.

Self-disclosure is never forced. Participants need to feel free not to reveal themselves if they so desire (which is really another norm in itself). One way that the leader can encourage self-disclosure is by revealing herself, which can be tricky because the timing must be rather precise. Early in the group's life an important issue is the leader's credibility. By revealing some of her own guilty secrets too soon she might sacrifice her credibility. Self-disclosure by the leader can be very helpful for the group because it helps dispel the authority issue. Clients can see that professionals are human and sometimes need the help that they can provide. I am, however, very loathe to self-disclose early in the life of the group, and hope that the self-disclosure norm will develop spontaneously from the emotional need for validation and from the trust and acceptance norms that begin to develop.

Confrontation Norm. It is vital that the group members learn to "check out" with one another when they are concerned about something. Many problems in interpersonal relationships occur as a result of assumptions that are made without any checks on reality. For example, the student who assumed I was angry with her because I did not smile when we met could operate on that assumption to the detriment of our relationship. If, however, we established a confrontation norm then the student would feel free to question me on how I feel about her and might find that I have been preoccupied with some personal problems and that my not smiling was not a reflection on how I feel about her. It might also come to pass that I was angry with her, and then we would have an opportunity to discuss that which is interfering in our relationship. In either event, we would both win from the confrontation.

I can relax in a group once a confrontation norm has been established because it means that my behavior and statements will not be misunderstood or go by unquestioned: the participants will test reality with me and with each other if need be.

The confrontation norm is best established by role modeling. The leader must pick an appropriate time to demonstrate this behavior. Confrontation requires a great deal of group trust and is frightening to members. Unfortunately, it is not common in many interpersonal relationships, and participants are usually fearful. Confrontation is closely related to self-disclosure because all confrontation involves a disclosure of self in regard to another person within the group. Self-disclosure emerges first because it is safer to talk about yourself than it is to talk about yourself in relationship to someone else who is present. The same conditions that will lead a group to self-disclosure will also lead to developing a confrontation norm.

Confrontation is not necessarily about negative feelings; one can also confront others with feelings of warmth and liking. I find, however, that the first confrontation feelings to emerge are very often anger and resentment. Most people are less threatened by expressing angry feelings than they are by expressing loving feelings. I find this fact very sad.

Here-and-Now Norm. Probably nothing is deadlier in a group than having members tell long anecdotes that nobody else has access to; interest in the group diminishes rapidly. I, as facilitator, have to find immediacy in the material and bring it to the present. Thus a participant who is relating a story in which she had a dispute with the hearing-aid dealer, for example, might get a response from me of "What did you do with your anger?" (invites self-disclosure) and then, "Have you been angry with me?" (invites confrontation). The more immediate the experience is the more exciting it is, and the greater the potential for it being a learning experience for everyone. When it is material that everyone has access to, as in recalling an event that happened in one of the group meetings, everyone can contribute and receive and give feedback.

A here-and-now norm is established by timely interventions on the facilitator's part, which force the group member into the present and immediate. Groups will not start out with a here-and-now orientation as they have no group history to work from. Participants have to reveal themselves and establish their credibility. There also needs to be some elapsed time for interactions among members to be processed. Here-and-now is a powerful norm directed toward achieving the goals of personal growth because it encourages interpersonal interaction within the group.

Respecting Individual Needs. Group norms, if not watched, can become very restrictive, especially when they promote a high degree of conformity. It is not healthy for everyone to adhere rigidly to a particular norm that is established. Individuals need to feel that they have control over their own behaviors, that learning will proceed when they are ready. One of the few explicit norms I establish in every group I lead is that the participants do not have to talk if they do not wish to, and that no question must be answered. When a group decision is required for a procedure it is necessary to arrive at a compromise or a willingness for the dissenters to agree to conform to the norm. For example, I cannot tolerate being in rooms in which there is a lot of cigarette smoke and I prefer that there be no smoking in the group. I tell this to the group at our first session and then talk to the smokers. I try to respect their felt "need" to smoke and see if they are willing to go the length of the session without smoking. If not, I offer a smoking break to the group in which we all stop for several minutes. If the room is especially well ventilated, I might agree to a limited amount of cigarettes being smoked during the session.

My willingness to negotiate and to discuss the issue with the smokers sends an important message to the group that I will try to respect each individual's needs. If I had come into the group with the statement that smoking is not permitted, I would be establishing a leader-dominated group in which my needs superseded other members' needs, and one in which I alone determined and imposed my needs on the group.

The time taken to negotiate the smoking issue is well spent; it establishes a powerful group norm. On such seemingly little things the success of the group depends.

Procedural Norms. There are norms that determine how the group will function. There are usually a number of givens in the situation that the group has no control over such as number of sessions and the length of time of each session. I am always very clear at the outset about how much time is available. If time is a negotiable issue with the group I will enter into negotiation that first session so that everyone knows what the length of their time commitment is and agrees to it. I also am sure to be at the group meeting on time and to end all meetings at the agreed upon hour.

I try to establish a norm of confidentiality in almost all counseling groups that I lead. I know I cannot impose confidentiality as I do not have any way of enforcing it. I tell the group that I will not talk about the group with any outsiders and that I hope they will do the same. I do not allow casual visitors to the group. In my academic classes, I do not talk about confidentiality in initial sessions because confidentiality implies (or almost imposes) a self-disclosure norm on a group. If a group of students begins to self-disclose I will then talk to them about confidentiality and see if we can come to some consensus.

STAGES OF GROUP DEVELOPMENT

While each group is unique, there seem to be some universals about group development, or at least all groups seem to develop along certain lines. The group facilitator needs to have a sense of the developmental sequence of groups to be able to diagnose quickly when a group is functioning deviantly and to perhaps provide some corrective measures. Almost invariably the difficulty will be caused by an unhealthy group norm, which is limiting group growth. There are virtually no controlled research studies on group development; what does exist is mainly nonsystematic clinical observations (Yalom, 1975).

The Group at Inception. I usually start groups by introducing myself, explaining how I came to be there and what expectations I have for myself in the group. I then invite each member to introduce herself and describe why she is there. After everyone has finished I mention any procedural norms (i.e., time of sessions, smoking, right to not answer questions, and so on). These are kept to a minimum as most norms are developed as a function of how I behave and which group behaviors I will reinforce. After speaking I might remark that I hope that everyone will come to value the experience. At this point usually a loud silence ensues, which seems to be eternal but is probably no more than 30 seconds in duration. Almost invariably the silence is broken by a question directed at me, which is usually a procedural-type question as the group begins to look to the leader to provide them with structure. For example, a participant might ask, "What are we supposed to do here?" (I usually respond, "What would you like to do here?")

The group at inception is characterized by developing structure and establishing credibility. When the members begin to learn that I will not structure the sessions they start to act, and in acting, reveal themselves. Everybody is still on their best "cocktail party" behavior; a parent group might begin by one telling the story about discovering her child's disability, which establishes credentials to be in the group, and invariably provokes other members to start telling their stories. When they find nods of acceptance and a matching of experiences, cohesiveness starts to build. Usually a lot of affect is expressed. The beginning stages of a parent group are usually very cathartic as they have all of the pent-up feelings that have not been expressed.

A student group or a working professional group usually starts out very hesitantly with long, embarrassed silences. The members are not sure how to proceed and are uncertain how much of themselves they are willing to reveal. Usually there is someone in the group who is desperate enough to risk some self-disclosure. If that is accepted, an intimacy spiral begins to develop, and more and more self-disclosures characterize the beginning stages.

Almost no confrontation occurs in beginning stages because there is not sufficient trust. Invariably confrontation stems from the leader's role-modeling this behavior, and it needs to occur at a somewhat later point in group development. A classic dilemma for the group leader occurs when there is a member of a beginning group who is starting to establish destructive norms for the group and no one is willing to confront her. For example, in a recent student group, one participant kept monopolizing the group with long, boring anecdotes that bore no relationship to what anyone else had been saying. She filled every silence, and commandeered the gaps between silences. No one in the group seemed confident enough to challenge her. I took responsibility for pointing out her behavior and solicited feedback from other members as to how they were feeling about her. My intervention came too soon in the group's development because the "monopolizer" started not attending; when she did attend she seldom spoke. She denied being fearful of speaking but seemed to lose all interest in the group. The rest of the group, however, became even more fearful, afraid that I might put them on the "hot seat." The group became a very low-risk, low-participation group characterized by long uncomfortable silences and very little self-disclosure. They no longer saw me as a support. Even though I solicited feedback about how they felt about the incident and about me, the group never became cohesive.

In retrospect I realize that I needed to wait longer before confronting the monopolizer in this group; I did not allow the group time to learn to act cohesively. Groups need time to develop sufficient trust: familiarity breeds liking when we can get below the surface behavior. I have found it a mistake to try to push groups in the early stages of development—it is an unfolding process.

Resistance to the group process also begins to develop early. The resistance usually manifests itself by the focusing on differences among the members. The parent groups that I lead at Emerson College are composed of parents of young deaf children, parents of normally hearing children, student clinicians, and not infrequently a practicing clinician who wants to learn more about groups. The professionals and I meet after the group session to process the experience. Almost invariably the professionals and students have a low level of participation in the group. They feel that it is a parent group and they have little to contribute. As they get more comfortable they begin to see the commonalities between themselves and the parents, and frequently use the group as a valuable personal growth vehicle. We can always find a reason for not doing something.

The Working Group. The developmental stages of a group are rarely well demarcated. There is no single point at which a group announces that it is ready to move from the inception stage to the working stage. This stage is characterized by cohesiveness, by conflict, and by redefining the leader.

It might seem contradictory to say that the group is cohesive as well as in conflict but these attributes are not incompatible. Only when an individual feels safe within a relationship can she afford to be confrontational. Conflict, when it emerges within the group, is usually a marker of the level of cohesiveness within the group. In initial stages everyone is on his or her best behavior, uncertain as to the safety of the situation. When the members feel secure, they confront. Usually the confrontation is with an outsider as when parents accuse the students of not having a child and therefore not being able to understand them. If no obvious outsider exists then the behavior is directed toward the leader for somehow failing them. (The leader in one sense is always an outsider and very often being group facilitator means that the leader has to continually confront her existential aloneness.)

At this point the group is ready to redefine the leader and to settle into its working structure. Anger is directed toward me because I will not tell them what to do, and parents wonder if I could possibly understand them as I do not have a disabled child. Conflict cannot be eliminated from human interaction; we grow from conflict. It is the resolution of the conflict that determines the group structure. We negotiate among ourselves, we compromise, and we develop the mechanisms that enable us to attend to tasks.

Content also becomes very valuable and is readily transferred among the members. A good working group is characterized by a joint knowledge of the strengths and weaknesses of each member and an ability to utilize the talent that is in the group. The topics that appeared in the initial stages of the group now reappear and are discussed in more detail and from a different perspective. Thus some participants who said little the first time around may become very vocal (the previous discussion may have set them to thinking about the issue and they are now ready to share). Other members may have rethought their positions. I find with parent groups in particular that all the cogent issues emerge in the first few sessions and no new topics occur thereafter. It is a recycling process. A richness and complexity are generated by the interactions of the group members, and groups never run out of things to say.

In a well-functioning group, the trust level is high, and when conflict does emerge it is dealt with openly. Positive feelings among the members emerge, and some are even directed toward the leader. She is now accepted as a working member of the group. I realize I am portraying an idealized vision of the working group. Not all of the groups I have dealt with achieve this level of functioning—many get close. Unfortunately some groups never get close. I have never yet failed to learn from a group.

The Terminating Group. Termination is an integral part of the group process and is not to be trivialized or minimized. The process of termination itself becomes an impetus to further growth. My own particular death avoidance issues very often interfered with providing the group a satisfactory termination ritual. Groups need time and space to tie up loose ends (there are always loose ends) and to mourn their demise. Often the group avoids the task of termination because it is a very painful task. The leader can use that termination awareness as a spur to complete work. I try to keep groups working until the last possible moment. Often groups will start the termination process too soon and if I allow this to happen we could lose some good work. It is a timing judgment that the leader must exercise.

I have come to terminate groups by suggesting that each member take a moment to reflect on the group experience and to imagine herself going home. "What messages do you wish you had delivered?" "What 'I should have saids' do you think you might have?" I then suggest that we spend the rest of the session delivering the messages. Yalom (1975) has the following to say about the termination process:

Throughout, the therapist facilitates the group work by disclosing his own feelings about separation. The therapist, no less than the patients, will miss the group. For him, too, it has been a place of anguish, conflict, fear, and also of great beauty; some of life's truest and most poignant moments occur in the small and yet limitless microcosm of the therapy group (p. 374).

OTHER CONSIDERATIONS

Use of Structured Experiences. Structured experiences are generally any activities, usually leader generated, that are designed to accelerate the group process. They are techniques that encourage self-disclosure or bypass the conventional social restrictions, for example, having a new group divide into dyads and having each member of the dyad interview the other. When the group reconvenes, each member of the dyad introduces the other to the group. There are many such devices to get through the initial introductory stage.

The problem with leader-directed exercises is that they do not encourage initiative by the group members. They tend to create a passive group, which sits back and waits for the leader to give the next exercise. The exercises can become an excuse for an individual's behavior and can limit responsibility assumption. Exercises frequently are used to rescue a group (actually, the leader) and in the long term they are seldom helpful to the group. Lieberman and colleagues (1973) found that group leaders who used exercises most frequently were regarded by the members of their groups as more competent, more effective, and more perceptive than leaders who used structured experiences sparingly. Yet, and very much to the point, the members of the highly structured experience groups had the poorest outcomes (i.e., less positive changes and less able to maintain positive change over time) than the low exercise group.

I have used and still occasionally use structured experiences in my workshops. I use them sparingly and they need to fit organically within the flow of the group process. When effective, they occur or seem to occur spontaneously. In my previous book (Luterman, 1979) I devoted an entire chapter to structured experience. These activities included role-playing, hypothetical families, and guided fantasies. Although I have had positive feedback from readers who have used them to advantage, I am always a bit uncomfortable with them and their use as I feel they can get a group and group leader into trouble that they may not yet be prepared to handle. Structured experiences can open members of a group sooner than a group is ready for it. They also seem to encourage a technique orientation for the group leader that I do not like.

I think structured experiences can be valuable if used judiciously. The interested reader is referred to material in my previous book, which can be adapted to any communication disorder.

Homogeneity of Grouping. The general tendency to keep groups homogeneous is usually reflected in the diagnostic label. Thus we have groups of laryngectomized persons, stutterers, families of stroke victims, and so on. When I began working with groups I restricted the group to parents of young, deaf children who were otherwise normal. I was trying for a very homogeneous group as I did not feel secure enough at that time to handle any additional problems presented by deviant parents. I soon learned that homogeneity is a myth. Even though the group shared the same diagnostic label there were enormous differences between and among the members. There were differences in education, values, and child-rearing practices. In fact, an early manifestation of resistance to the group process was the pointing out of the many differences that existed between the members (e.g., "They can't possibly understand me because I stutter and they do not," and so on). One of the primary tasks of the facilitator is to focus the group on their similarities ("Can you tell me some ways in which you are like these other people?").

As I have become more secure in my abilities I have allowed more obvious heterogeneous groupings to occur. I began letting parents of multiply-disabled, hearing-impaired children into the group, parents of older deaf children, and parents of normally hearing children. Recently, I have worked with groups of parents of children of mixed disabilities. Each time I have increased the apparent heterogeneity of the group, the group has become richer for it. Parents of hearing children have added a commonality to the child-rearing problems, parents of older deaf children have added their experience, while parents of other disabled children have led to the appreciation of the universality of the experience of parenting a handicapped child. These different parents have stretched me professionally, and I now welcome and encourage diversity in my groups.

Group Size and Setting. Generally the groups I work with are between 8 and 15 members. I find that this is a good working group size because there are enough members for sufficient interactions among the participants, and not so many as to require inordinate amounts of time for members to establish their credibility. Larger groups take much longer to establish trust. I also do not allow new people to join the group except at clearly marked demarcation points such as semester breaks. New members tend to hold back the group development as the group requires time to absorb the newcomer and to reestablish cohesiveness. It also takes a while for the new member to figure out the group norms.

I always try to hold meetings in a comfortable room and to have the participants sitting in a circle. In this way members can establish eye contact with each other and can read each other's body language (so can the leader). Chairs also need to be comfortable as the duration of most groups is 1 to 2 hours. A professor of mine once said that the mind can absorb only as much as the seat can endure.

Filling the Available Time. The duration of a group is usually arbitrarily determined. The exigencies of calendar, finances, and participant availability seem to have more bearing on group length than does amount of therapeutic progress. In one sense, groups are never finished; they are always in the process of becoming and new material is always emerging. In this way they are not unlike human beings. For me, the group meeting is a magical moment to be enjoyed and savored for that time and never to be replicated.

Groups have a marvelous way of filling the available time. There is a subconscious and I think collective knowledge as to how far we can go together on our journey. Rogers was once asked, "How far can you get with nondirective therapy when you have only 20 minutes' time?" His response was "20 minutes' worth." I have had some wonderfully intense group experiences where the total duration of the group was 2 hours. These groups are almost like a speeded-up motion picture: we all know that we have only 2 hours to work, all of the trivialities are eliminated, cohesiveness develops very quickly, and self-disclosure becomes high. Several of my most satisfying professional experiences have occurred in groups with a very short life span.

The counseling group can have a tremendous value in the therapeutic process. It can be used for the families of communicatively disordered individuals as a supplement to individual therapy, or it can be combined into therapy and counseling sessions.

Groups can be used very flexibly, and developing skills in facilitating groups should be part of a speech-language therapist's training.

B I B L I O G R A P H Y

Albertini, J., Smith, J., and Metz, D. Small group versus individual speech therapy with hearing impaired young adults. *Volta Rev.* 85:83, 1983.

Backus, O., and Beasley, J. *Speech Therapy with Children.* Cambridge, Mass.: Houghton Mifflin, 1951.

Bardach, J. Group sessions with wives of aphasic patients. *Int. J. Group Psychother.* 119:361, 1969.

Dee, A. Meeting the needs of the parents of deaf infants: A comprehensive parent-education program. *Language, Speech and Hearing Services in Schools* 12:13, 1981.

Emerson, R. *Changes in Depression and Self-Esteem of Spouses of Stroke Patients with Aphasia as a Result of Group Counseling.* Ph.D. dissertation. Oregon University, 1980.

Lieberman, M., Yalom, I., and Miles, M. *Encounter Groups: First Facts.* New York: Basic Books, 1973.

Luterman, D. *Counseling Parents of Hearing Impaired Children.* Boston: Little, Brown, 1979.

Schein, J. Group techniques applied to deaf and hearing-impaired persons. In M. Seligman, *Group Psychotherapy and Counseling with Special Populations.* Baltimore: University Park Press, 1982.

Seligman, M. *Group Psychotherapy and Counseling with Special Populations.* Baltimore: University Park Press, 1982.

Singler, J. The Stroke Group: Planning for Success. In M. Seligman, *Group Psychotherapy and Counseling with Special Populations.* Baltimore: University Park Press, 1982.

Webster, E. Procedures for group counseling in speech pathology and audiology. *J. Speech Hear. Disord.* 33:27, 1968.

Webster, E. *Counseling with Parents of Handicapped Children.* New York: Grune & Stratton, 1977.

Yalom, I. *The Theory and Practice of Group Psychotherapy.* New York: Basic Books, 1975.

CHAPTER 6

PARENT-PROFESSIONAL

RELATIONSHIP

Parent education is almost synonymous with motherhood and the American way of life—that is, almost no one speaks against it. At meeting after meeting, speakers affirm in the most solemn tones how important parents are; yet the practice of parent education, in my opinion, leaves much to be desired.

PROFESSIONALS

Professional Attitudes. Perhaps representative of parent education programs within the field of communication disorders is the program described by Dee (1981) for hearing parents of deaf children. An important component of this early intervention program was weekly sessions with parents. Content generally was provided by the professionals on topics that were generated by the parents, who were required to bring notebooks to each session. Dee also stressed the need for the professional to be sensitive to the emotional needs of the parents, and for the professional to be a nonjudgmental listener (although it is not at all clear within her description when any affect counseling was to take place). The attitude that Dee has toward parents is, I think, reflected in a section of the article titled "The role of parent education in developing and sustaining positive parental attitudes toward total communication."

Most hearing parents of deaf infants need considerable help and guidance in developing clear and honest convictions about the real values of the total communication approach in the life of a deaf infant and his/her family. Even after their first pleasurable experience with total communication during family sessions, when they have learned how to achieve a warm and loving communication interaction with their infant, some of our parents will continue to undergo periods of doubt, uncertainty, and even occasional resistance. Parents might also be struggling against non-supportive and/or antagonistic attitudes towards manual communication expressed by grandparents, relatives, friends. Furthermore, almost all parents cannot help but be vulnerable to the highly persuasive claims of the oralists. It is essential, therefore, to provide parents in total communication programs with a strong and convincing rationale for continuing to use this communication mode. A parent education program can provide year-long opportunities for exploring and evaluating all that is "total" about total communication and for expanding and strengthening parental understanding of and belief in the emotional and educational gains that are the rewards of a total communication way of life (p. 15).

This article could have very easily been written by someone from the "oralist" school. The ensuing discussion is not in any way meant as an indictment of total communication, only of this particular kind of parent education.

The underlying assumptions of this type of education are that parents are weak and cannot be trusted to make the right decision. It also assumes that the professional knows best and has the responsibility to tell (or even coerce) parents into the right behavior and thinking. Actually this approach to parent education fosters a belief system; it will tend to create unthinking parents.

Dee's ideas are not education as I see it. Education should leave people with confidence in their ability to make their own decisions. They also must take responsibility for those decisions. The result of Dee's program will leave the parents either very dependent on the professionals for the "right answer" or, suspecting a sales pitch, will leave them very suspicious about all professionals and their particular axe to grind. In either case, it is not a healthy attitude and does not reflect any personal growth or a healthy parent-professional relationship. Unfortunately, I see many programs of parent education built along these doctrinaire lines, which create fanatic and dependent parents, not well-educated or self-confident ones.

Professional Training. I think that the failure of adequate parent programs is a reflection of the failure at the training level to provide good models of parent programming. Cartwright and Ruscello (1979) surveyed all 134 programs, which up to that time were certified by the American Board of Examiners in Speech Pathology and Audiology, on the extent of parent involvement in their programs. Of the 115 returned questionnaires, they found that 89 percent of the respondents considered parent involvement an essential part of their services. Despite this statement, only 51 percent of the clinics had any organized parent program. I think this result reflects the "schizophrenia" of our field regarding parent education. The vast majority of professionals feel that parents are important, yet only half of the facilities have any organized program. Those programs responsible for the training of students reported higher percentage of organized parent programs (66%), although of these programs only 17 percent required students to enroll in courses dealing with parent involvement. In many programs informal parent training was at the discretion of individual supervisors. Moreover, the American Speech-Language and Hearing Association (ASHA) does not recognize practicuum hours of parent involvement in student training—only direct-care contact. (This attitude is true also for many job descriptions of working speech-language pathologists whereby they are only allowed to count direct contact hours with the client toward their remuneration; any other hours of family contact are at the clinician's discretion. No wonder there is so little parent involvement.) Because parent contact is not mandated by ASHA, one wonders how many students leave training programs without any parent involvement even when there is a parent program available.

I think it a fair statement that many speech-language pathologists and audiologists leave their respective training programs with a minimum of involvement with parents. In addition, they are invariably (at least when they start) younger than the parents and many are not parents themselves and consequently often feel insecure and defensive. Student trainees in our nursery program often talk about how uncomfortable they are dealing with young deaf children while the parents can see them. They are afraid that they will do something that the parent will not approve of, and that they will somehow offend the parent. The students are invariably much more afraid of being with the parents than they are of being with the children.

The professional insecurity manifests itself in a variety of ways. In many clinics, for example, one sees the parents in the waiting room while the child is having therapy with the professional. I think the most prevalent manifestation is that of keeping the relationship in the content areas. As long as the professional can lecture and tell parents what to do, he can control the relationship. It helps no end if the professional requires parents to bring a notebook. This, as it does with students, automatically confers a superior status on the teacher and an inferior one on the learner. I can also see many distancing strategies determined by dress and title, all of which are taught to the student in training as being professional. This notion of being a professional is in actuality an armor designed to protect the neophyte clinician from exposing his insecurity. Unfortunately, the behavior persists long after the trainee passes the insecure stage, and many veteran speech pathologists and audiologists still have very personally distant, nonintimate relationships with parents under the guise of professionalism.

Another personality factor that seems to limit the openness of parent-professional relationships is the strong need to be needed, which is exhibited by many professionals in the helping professions. When the professional is using the children to fulfill some personal holes left from his own deprivations, then the parent, albeit on a subconscious basis, is really a competitor for the child's affection. Although the professional may voice concern about involving parents more, in reality he wishes to prove that he is the better parent. This I call the Annie Sullivan syndrome (see Chap. 2). Annie's returning from the shack with a now tractable child after just a week demonstrated to Mrs. Keller her inadequacies, and because she loved Helen, she began to feel that Helen would be better off with Annie. Mrs. Keller became reduced to the role of a loving aunt (i.e., she was involved in decisions regarding Helen's welfare, but she never seemed to assume any active mothering role after Annie came on the scene).

Again, Helen Keller's case is an extreme example, but I think variations of the competition between parent and teacher for the child are frequently played out in therapy, and it is necessary for professionals to have their personal needs met outside of their work experience.

The professional insecurity engendered by limited training in parent education, a nontrusting attitude toward parents, and a competitive stance regarding the child have, I believe, limited good parent–professional programming from the professional side of the equation. The onus is not, however, entirely on the professional. The parent brings to the relationship many negative feelings and behaviors, which make it difficult for a good relationship to be established.

P A R E N T S

Parental Inadequacy. Parents of handicapped children feel overwhelmed and generally very inadequate at parenting. Any parent who is willing to be introspective about the task recognizes that raising an infant to adulthood is an awesome responsibility. When they are told that the child is handicapped and given the inspirational speech by the professional that begins "If this child is to succeed it is up to you. . .," the parents feel even more inadequate. These feelings of inadequacy usually manifest themselves in trying to find someone who will rescue them, in short, trying to find an Annie Sullivan. The parents also saw the movie *The Miracle Worker*, and a frequent fantasy discussed in the parent groups is the "wouldn't it be nice if someone came and took my child now and brought him back when he was 18—all civilized and talking beautifully" dream. This fantasy is usually talked about with a laugh but does reflect the underlying insecurity and feelings of inadequacy felt by the parents.

In one parent group a father wanted me to be the quarterback of his team. When I declined he offered me the position of coach, which I also declined. The only role in his personal odyssey that I was willing to accept was that of enthusiastic fan. I told him that I would be in the stands rooting hard and sharing all my information, but that he would have to send in his own plays. Unfortunately, too many professionals are willing to be the quarterback. When the professional calls the plays, the parents become the spectators and assume no responsibility for the outcome. They may either praise the players or blame them but they are not involved. Spectators seldom grow or learn very much.

Parental Anger. Parents of handicapped children are angry. At some very basic level, having a handicapped child engenders anger. One source of the anger is the loss of control over their lives. Parents feel that they can no longer operate in their own best interest—having a handicapped child means losing degrees of personal freedom. Fathers have to give up promotions because the new towns have no programs for deaf children; mothers who were planning to return to work now have to defer it because they feel needed at home to provide added stimulation for their handicapped children; families that have to move from very desirable locations to be nearer educational facilities for the handicapped child are all examples of the loss of control. It is very easy for parents to feel resentment at having to make these changes, which are imposed from outside and over which they have little or no control.

Another source of anger is the violation of expectation. If you and I have an agreement to meet and you fail to show up at the appointed time, I will be very angry; it is a self-righteous anger. Parents have many expectations about their own unborn child;

the major one is that he will be normal. When the child is not normal, the parents get very angry. They feel cheated. Another expectation, frequently doomed to failure, is that the disorder can be cured. Parents find it harder to accept the fact that there is no cure than to accept the fact of their child being disabled. ("We spend so much money to send an astronaut to the moon — why can't we find a cure for cerebral palsy?") They also have expectations of the professional and usually expect to be taken care of and told what to do; this expectation may or may not be violated.

The most pervasive and perhaps most harmful expectation is what parents expect of themselves. In my experience many parents have very high expectations of their own coping abilities. They often see it as a weakness when they cry and when they cannot absorb all the information thrown at them. They despair because they despair and because they are, at times, incompetent in dealing with their child's problems. This anger becomes directed at themselves and manifests itself in low self-esteem and frequently in depression. Parents (and professionals) need to learn to give themselves permission to be incompetent at times.

Another feeling, which is more like rage, is born of the frustration of having a child who is hurt in some way and not being able to do anything about it. All parents are pledged to make things better for their child, and when they are powerless to do so they experience rage. It is a rage born of impotence.

I think most professionals intuitively recognize that they are dealing with angry people when they are with parents, and, in part, many of the distancing strategies are self-protection from the parental anger. Very often the parental anger at the situation is displaced onto the professional, and the professional can very easily become the lightning rod. Many times people slay the messenger when they do not like the message.

Anger can be a very healthy emotion in relationships. There is a great deal of caring and energy in anger. If parents are angry at me I examine the anger to see if it is justified. If I have been derelict in my duty, I apologize and make amends if possible. If we are dealing with a situation in which there has been an implicit expectation that I have failed to meet, the anger then becomes an opportunity to clarify our relationship and to make the expectation explicit. If I am dealing with displaced anger, then we can clarify and start to direct the anger into more useful channels as, for example, working to help other parents of handicapped children or educating the public and physicians about the problems of the communicatively disordered. There is never any loss in dealing openly and honestly with anger. It took me a long time to recognize that, as I had always thought that anger was equated with loss of love.

When anger is subverted and not allowed to emerge, it poisons relationships. People who are angry with me and do not tell me frequently operate in subversive ways. Thus is born the parent who chronically misses appointments, is bothered by very minor things such as the decor of the room or the comfort of the chairs, and who does not fully participate in the program. Unless I can tap into the anger and deal with it, our relationship will never be mutually satisfactory. Professionals very often feel that they do not have the right to be angry at parents, and they will repress or displace their anger to the detriment of their relationship. Unexpressed anger is like a loaded cannon loose on deck, which can go off at any moment and sink the vessel.

Anger will not emerge unless there is a high degree of trust and intimacy in a relationship. Only secure people can afford to risk the loss of relationship by showing anger. Relationships are almost always strengthened after anger emerges if it is dealt with openly. The professional needs to be secure in himself as a person and needs to be working very hard on establishing trust in relationships so as to allow any anger to emerge—then the relationship can withstand and grow from controversy.

Parental Guilt. The feeling of guilt that almost all parents (especially mothers) have often muddies the parent-professional relationship. Guilt arises very often out of the parents' religious experiences, and (as was discussed in Chap. 2) parents often see their handicapped child as a punishment for some sin that they committed. It is almost impossible to lead such a blameless life that you cannot find a reason for the wrath of God to be visited on you. Even if you cannot find the sin, God must have found it.

With many congenital disorders, the cause is unknown and parents frequently will look back on the pregnancy to find a cause. Very often the search for the cause is a reflection of the guilt feelings. Parents want to be absolved of their guilt and hope to find a cause that they can in no way be responsible for. Unfortunately, many times the cause cannot be determined and parents are forced to reflect on their own experience. Many mothers "know" that they caused the handicap by not taking vitamin pills when they were supposed to or by not following completely some direction of the physician. Although most of these guilty secrets are unfounded and cannot stand examination, a trusting, intimate relationship must be established in which the parent feels free to talk about this "awful thing" she has done to cause her child's handicap. The unconditional regard of the professional will help parents to reveal the guilty secret. We can probably bestow no greater gift than to relieve a parent of unfounded guilt.

Most parents are driven by their guilty feelings, and the consequences of guilt are usually not very wholesome for the family. Guilty parents tend to overprotect their child, their reasoning being that: "we let something bad happen to you once and we are not about to allow it to happen to you again." These parents will not let their child develop much autonomy or initiative. They will seldom let the child out of their sight and will be uncomfortable when they do. The overprotection will extend to the therapy situation; these parents are not very trusting of the professionals and of professional competency, questioning the therapist and frequently seeking other opinions. It is very hard to maintain a long-term relationship with a guilt-driven parent.

Guilt feelings also lead to the "superdedicated" parent, often the mother. This parent reasons that "I let something bad happen to you and now I am going to make it up to you." This parent often fools professionals in the preschool years because she looks so good—doing lessons with the child and doing much more than anyone could reasonably expect. This cost is very high, usually in terms of the family. The husband-wife relationship is strained by the absentee parent and the other siblings also suffer from the diminished attention. The biggest damage is probably inflicted on the parent herself. With such dedication there is little or no room to develop any other aspects of her potential and she has a limited identity outside of being the "parent of a handicapped child." Although these parents look very good in the preschool years when their dedication is usually reflected in highly achieving youngsters, they look very bad when they are parents of adolescent children and must let go of the child. At this point they frequently need the child to define themselves: to let go would mean a huge identity crisis. Parents often need a great deal of help when their children reach adolescence, not only in managing the child but in managing their own feelings and anxieties.

Guilt is such an uncomfortable feeling. It gives rise to resentment, but unlike anger resentment seldom if ever is expressed directly, and relationships that are built on guilt are seldom healthy. Unfortunately, many parent-child, parent-parent, and parent-professional relationships have a high guilt component, and consequently do not grow.

I have never yet met a mother of a deaf child who wanted to have a deaf child or deliberately set about causing deafness in her child. The discussion of guilt emerges in almost all parent groups. When the parent was directly responsible through some dereliction of duty, I try to help establish an expiation contract ("I will pay back by doing such and such, and then I can leave my guilt alone"). Where it is a guilt built on ignorance, such as thinking that failure to take a vitamin pill causes deafness, information can help alleviate the painful feelings. Where it is a neurotic guilt, as it seems to be in many cases, then a group discussion among parents seems to help as well as all the personal growth opportunities provided within the program. In any event, a major goal of counseling should be the disengagement of the guilty feelings from the nonproductive behavior. Parents can feel guilty and still behave in a self-enhancing way.

Parental Confusion. Almost all parents as they go through the learning process are confused. Confusion is a normal stage when we attempt to acquire new information that we do not have a background to evaluate or when we are unfamiliar with the vocabulary. The professional can contribute to the parental confusion by having a content-based relationship with the parent.

Professionals often forget how difficult it was for them to acquire the vocabulary of their profession, otherwise known as jargon. Such terms as *audiologist*, *language* (as opposed to speech), *speech pathologist* are fairly esoteric terms to most people, yet we bandy these about with parents. We might define the term once and then assume it is understood. We forget that learning takes time and patience.

For me, content was the prime distancing strategy. If I kept our relationship on content (which also met both the parents' and my expectations) then I could be in control and we did not need to tap into the grief and anger, which I did not know how to deal with. This strategy severely limits the relationship and increases the confusion period by providing the parents with too much gratuitous information. The professional is not the only source of information, however. Parents are receiving information from many different places, and much of it, especially in the field of deafness with its many controversies, is conflicting.

The parent-professional relationship can be used as a place where the parents get a chance to sort out the information received and to come to some conclusion for themselves. In order for this to happen the professional needs to be very judicious about supplying information. The professional can supply information (not opinion) when needed. As a general rule of thumb I do not give parents information unless they ask for it. I will generally ask them, "What do you need to know?" When I receive as a response "I don't even know enough to ask a question," which is not atypical in the very early stages, I might respond, "It sounds like you are pretty confused," and we can start talking about this confusion. This opening often becomes an invitation to discuss their affect surrounding the child's handicap. The content questions and answers will come later.

When the parents ask specific content questions, I try to answer with the content. I would like to think that my answers are opinion free but I have, like most professionals in this field, strong opinions. The best I can do is identify them for the parents and label them as opinion. There is a need and a place for content during the initial stages of relationship; it fulfills an implicit contract between professionals and their client population. Information also helps to establish credibility, and my own feeling is that in the initial stages the information functions more to establish credibility than to alleviate ignorance. Parental feelings are turbulent and parents are very confused; thus, that little of what is said to them is retained. Frequently, parents, when they try to recall their initial contact with the audiologist, can remember some insignificant detail such as "I remember her dress had a blue checked pattern, but I can't remember anything she said." What parents do retain is the feeling of the relationship, whether or not the audiologist seemed to care. The caring came across as someone who listened and gave them time. Parents are invariably "turned off" by professionals who use the time to tell the parents everything they should do and who hurry them.

Parental Denial. Probably no single factor impairs parent-professional relationships as much as the denial mechanism. Denial must be seen by the professional for what it is, namely, a coping strategy based on feelings of inadequacy. Denial is a very normal and a very human reaction, which occurs in all of us. When I am driving my car, for example, and the engine begins to sound strange, I respond by putting on the radio. If the engine noises get louder, I increase the loudness of the radio. I know cognitively that putting on the radio is not going to solve my problem, but at that time, psychologically it is the only thing I can do. In short, I try to deny the existence of the problem, hoping that it will go away by itself. My need to adopt the radio strategy is based on my lack of confidence in my ability to repair engines. I feel totally inadequate around things mechanical—certainly anything as complicated as a car engine. If you were to admonish me about how silly I am to respond by putting on the radio I would grin sheepishly and agree with you. However, if I have no other strategy for coping with engine failure, then, when you are not around, I will use it.

Unless I am given other ways of coping, and gain some confidence in myself, I cannot afford to give up denial. If, for example, I had a course in engine maintenance, which I passed, then I would hear the slightest noise and pull the car over to the side of the road, coping with the crisis in a more responsible way than denying its existence.

Denial for the parent of a handicapped child is a coping mechanism that occurs at all levels. (Denial, of course, is not a mechanism restricted solely to parents. It is used by all disabled populations and will occur in almost all clients seen by the speech and language pathologist and audiologist.) Anytime there is a new demand on parental resources, when they are going to have to be wise or strong, denial will begin to operate. The most obvious time is at diagnosis. Very often the delay in getting a child diagnosed is because the parents cannot get themselves to admit that something may be wrong. Often, however, it is not solely the strategy of the parent; others in the environment practice denial, especially grandparents, and one even finds this mechanism operating in professionals, mainly the family pediatrician.

Denial persists at the habilitating level even when the parents freely acknowledge that they have a handicapped child. In deafness, denial will occur around anything that will objectify the deafness. The hearing aid, for example, becomes a powerful reminder that the child is deaf. Parents hate to see it on their child even though they know it helps the child. When they take pictures of the child they remove the hearing aid. When they send the child to school, the hearing aid is under several layers of clothing and, when uncovered, found to be nonfunctional. If the parents are in a total communication program, the denial can become focused on the signing; thus we have a parent who never attends class or, when he does, cannot seem to learn how to sign.

The professional, who is child-centered, sees the parental denial as an impediment to the child's progress (which it is) and gets angry at the parents. If the professional is direct about the anger, this results in an admonitory lecture about how important it is for the child to wear the aid or how necessary it is for the parents to attend signing class. The parents will grin sheepishly and agree with the professional (they knew how important it was before the professional told them) but because they have no other coping strategy (much as I didn't with my car) they will fall back on denial. After an initial period of attendance at classes or increased hearing-aid use, they will revert to denial, which will then provoke another round of professional ire.

The professional must learn to see the denial as a plea for help, and not as a dereliction of duty on the parents' part. No parents, at least those that I have met, want to do badly by their child. It is just that so many of the fears get in the way of their operating constructively. People cannot be pushed out of denial. They will give it up when they feel confident that they can be more successful with some other strategy. Denial may be the only way that the parents can cope with the current situation. Denial is an invitation to talk about feelings of inadequacy. By listening and by indirect teaching, which does not deskill them (diminish their feelings of competency), parents can be taught some fruitful coping strategies. If the professional is geared toward the child and is anxious about the child's welfare, then parental denial might provoke an adversarial relationship with the parents, which destroys any productive counseling relationship. Professionals very often try to "save" the child from the parent. Short of removing the child from the home, this cannot be done. Children cannot be saved from their parents—all of us, in one sense, are victims of our parents' failings. The professional must not let the parental denial impair the development of a healthy relationship.

The identification of behavior as denial is very tricky. It is not always clear when the parents are denying or when there is a legitimate difference of opinion between parents and professional. For example, in Chapter 4, Johnny was diagnosed by the staff as being a multihandicapped child. When the mother refused to accept that diagnosis we labeled her as a denying parent and tried to get her to see Johnny our way. She subsequently proved to be correct. Denial can be used to try to substitute professional "truth" for parental "truth"—and room must be allowed for a difference of opinion.

One person's denial may be another person's optimism. Frequently, when the professional has a very pessimistic prognosis for a child, the parent keeps saying "He will make it." Children have a way of meeting expectations and when the expectations are negative, children seldom perform well. Too often I have seen the parents proved right, and there is never any need to diminish parental optimism so long as their behavior is consistent with expected management practices. The optimism frequently gets translated into hope and many parents have the "maybe someday they will find a cure" dream, which is very sustaining for them. The dream enables them to work vigorously in the present and sustains them when they despair. It should never be doused by the professional. There is probably no crueler act than to deprive the parents of this dream.

There is also much that is positive about denial. In 1962, the Federal Government declared Spanish-American War veterans, of which there were only several hundred in the United States, totally disabled. This declaration entitled them to receive full benefits at the Veterans' Administration and also occasioned the launching of a large-scale study of the aged male. These men were in their eighties at the time and the study involved gathering data on all aspects of their life. I was involved in studying their hearing. As part of the examination I would interview them about how well they thought they could hear. This part of the research protocol became meaningless as everyone of them felt he could hear "fine" despite the fact that in many instances I had to shout in order to be heard. I spoke to the project psychologist about this phenomenon and he said it was pervasive throughout the study. These men persistently denied any infirmity and he concluded—only partially tongue in cheek—that perhaps one of the major secrets of living to a ripe old age is to assiduously practice denial.

Parental Vulnerability. Probably no one is more vulnerable than a parent when his child is involved. Having a disabled child dramatically increases parental vulnerability; so much more seems to be on the line for the parents. The parents think that they have to be operating at maximum capacity in order to develop their child's limited potential. They often think that this child is so delicately poised on the brink of failure that they cannot afford to make a mistake.

Professionals need to be very sensitive to this vulnerability. Sometimes a chance, off-hand remark by a professional can send the parent into the depths of despair or a paroxysm of joy. Professionals have an enormous amount of psychological power over parents whether they like it or not. All parents need to be approached with the loving concern that we would give to any sensitive human being in pain.

TRAINING STUDENTS FOR PARENT PROGRAMS

If there is going to be any meaningful change in the current parent-professional relationship it will have to occur at the professional training level. I think too many young clinicians leave their training programs with minimal or very inadequate experience in relating to parents. I suspect that part of the problem lies in the lack of practice in parent training of the supervisors and academic teachers in the training programs. ASHA can facilitate a growth in parent training by mandating that some of the clock hours required for certification be in parent involvement. If they do not mandate specific parent involvement hours, ASHA could at least allow the hours spent with parents to count toward certification. Cartwright and Ruscello (1979) suggest that 10 percent of the contact hours be allowed, which seems quite reasonable to me. On a national level, we also need to be promoting continuing education workshops specifically geared toward professionals in academic programs on the utilization of parents and the training of students in parent involvement.

We also need to look at our selection process for students. Currently we are selecting students on the basis of cognitive skills. We need to look at their emotional maturity as well. If possible, we need to build in more personal growth experiences for students at the training level. (See Chap. 8 for a further discussion of this issue.)

We need to increase the number and quality of our parent involvement programs throughout the nation. Only one-half of all approved clinics have a parent involvement program. This figure seems inadequate to me especially in light of the fact that nearly 90 percent of all programs feel that parent involvement is so important. We should also be very concerned about the quality of the parent programming. There are too many professional-centered parent programs (by this I mean programs in which the professional has the control and uses the educational program to promote a particular point of view) in which the personal growth of the parents is minimal.

Good parent programs have a snowball effect. They produce self-confident, positively assertive parents who will work as equals with other professionals. These parents, in effect, become trainers of other professionals. They open the eyes of professionals to the potential of parent involvement. What a relief it is, to a reasonably self-confident professional, to have a parent as a co-worker. Although these programs do exist, I would like to see them increase and it is to this end that this book was written.

If parent-professional relationships are to improve, they have to be freed from a problem-centered orientation. So much of the contact between parent and professional occurs only when there is a specific problem. It is very hard to have a productive relationship when it is always problem-centered. I give my aural rehabilitation class a role-playing situation in which a teacher of the deaf calls the parent to school to tell the parent that her child is "an oral failure" and should be put in a total communication program. The problem is set up to be adversarial in that the parent is strongly committed to an oral education. The situation usually ends up in disaster, in part because if this is the first parent-professional meeting (as generally happens) it is already too late. Time has not been spent in developing the necessary trust, autonomy, and initiative before they can get down to deal with such a loaded topic as changing the mode of communication for the child.

Some students solve the problem well by not projecting the problem onto the parent or child. They recognize that the person with the problem is the teacher. When the teacher can convey to the parents that she has a problem and can enlist the parents' help, then the relationship does not become adversarial. Both parents and teacher can embark together on a quest to find the best way of educating the child. It is also agreed by the class after the role-playing that the teacher should have seen the parents outside of the school and established and worked on their relationship before any problems occurred.

Parents and professional are natural allies. They both want in the most ardent terms the same thing: a better-communicating child. As Murphy (1981) in an almost lyrically written and lovely book on parents, *Special Children, Special Parents*, has written:

Parents and workers are sculptors helping to shape what a child may become. There is a place for all—a place to be, to become something more than they now are, a place to learn, to dance, to sing (p. ix).

BIBLIOGRAPHY

Cartwright, L., and Ruscello, D. A survey on parent involvement in speech clinics, *ASHA* 21:275, 1979.

Dee, A. Meeting the needs of the parents of deaf infants: A comprehensive parent-education program. *Language, Speech and Hearing Services in Schools* 12:13, 1981.

Murphy, A. *Special Children, Special Parents*. Englewood Cliffs, N.J.: Prentice-Hall, 1981.

CHAPTER 7

THE FAMILY

Probably the most pervasive influence on family therapy has been the work of Virginia Satir. Trained as a psychiatric social worker, she was assigned to the back wards of a mental hospital. She recognized early in her career that the traditional individual psychotherapeutic method of working with these patients was not effective. She began insisting that family members attend the counseling sessions. Gradually, as the family members began to interact with the identified patient, Satir realized that they seemed to have a stake in maintaining the patient as "sick." The family achieves a balance or homeostasis and adjusts to the person's illness (actually, it is the patient who may have responded to the family dynamics by being ill). As the patient attempts to recover, the family homeostasis is threatened and the tendency for the family is to maintain the person as ill. Satir (1967) found that as she worked with the family dynamics she was able to affect dramatic changes in the patients.

Families also attempt to maintain homeostasis when a disabled child is born into it or when a family member becomes disabled. Frequently, the denial mechanism is used to try to maintain homeostasis. When denial is challenged, it seems to the family members that their fundamental security is being threatened. Clinicians must be very sensitive and cautious in working with a family that is using denial to maintain homeostasis.

The concept of family homeostasis apparently has had some limited application in communication disorders. Egolf and colleagues (1972) found that working with young stutterers within the clinic was not sufficient to affect cures. They recommend that clinicians work with the parent–child dyad. As they put it,

If the child adjusts to his environment by stuttering, then the parent must have made an equal adjustment in maintaining stuttering—thus the dyad is in balance (equilibrium). If treatment changes one member of the dyad, the child, by making him fluent, the dyad is forced into disequilibrium. A new equilibrium requires changes in both parent and child (p. 223).

Clinicians must come to realize that the people we deal with are part of a system and that we cannot treat one element (the person with the communication disorder) without some attention to the entire system (the family). Robertson and Suinn (1968) found that there was a direct correlation between the empathy of family members and the recovery rate of stroke patients. Edgerly (1975) found that a program that provided parent education and tutoring yielded significantly more gains in academic achievement with learning disabled children than a regular curriculum program. He concluded "that parents must be directly involved in the treatment program if it is to be successful."

The Edgerly study, I think, demonstrates how efficacious family work is in effecting therapeutic progress. Aside from the experimental evidence, there is immense face validity in working with families. It seems incredibly presumptuous of therapists to think that if they spend 1 or 2 hours a week with a child they can change her speech or language behavior markedly. A much more effective use of therapeutic time would be to work to change the family dynamics and to make the home environment more conducive to growth. Yet, despite the logic of this rationale, there seems to be little direct family involvement in the communication disorders field. Probably the most family work is being done with congenitally deaf children (Elwood, Johnson, and Mandeld, 1977).

In this chapter we will examine two family situations: the family with a disabled child and the family in which a significant adult undergoes a traumatic illness. Both of these families will be under severe stress and the speech-language pathologist/audiologist can do a great deal to help alleviate some of that stress and thereby help the client.

THE FAMILY WITH A DISABLED CHILD

The initial reaction of the family to having a disabled child is a pulling together—a marshalling of the resources. As the parents begin to realize that the problem is long term, the chronic nature of the disability begins to wear at the parental unity. Featherstone (1980) notes that the child's disability strains the marriage. By evoking strong emotions in both parents, it becomes a fertile source of conflict and disrupts the organization of the family. On a long-term basis the disabled child is always a symbol of a shared failure.

Parents. The emotions involved in having a disabled child are very intense. Probably the most potentially maritally destructive emotion is anger. Because the parents usually have no satisfactory outlet for anger (many do not even recognize it and in others anger is repressed and emerges as depression) and in many families the expression of anger is not sanctioned, anger is often displaced. The parents may have a fight about the quality of the cooking or the whiteness of the laundry, which is way out of proportion to the "crime." A rule of thumb for me is that, in the early stages of diagnosis and therapy, what the parents are fighting about is seldom what they are really angry about. The loss of control, the impotence they feel in the face of their child's disability, fuels many a fight. Much of the anger is also displaced onto the professionals.

Guilt is another potentially destructive emotion to a marriage if it is not recognized and dealt with effectively. Guilt is usually felt by both parents although mothers, because they have carried the child during the pregnancy, seem to carry a heavier freight of guilt. Because guilt is such an uncomfortable feeling, the parents will try to push it off on each other. Thus begins the search through their family tree to find some defective relative, preferably on the spouse's side of the family. In combination with rage, guilt can be a formidable divisive force. The angry blaming that parents can fall into has split many a marriage.

With guilt often comes the "superdedicated" parent. This parent becomes committed to "making it up" to the disabled child, usually at the expense of the rest of the family. Less attention is paid to the husband-wife relationship and to the normal siblings. The parent very often ignores her own needs and becomes unidimensional—almost monomaniacal. The child's disability becomes the dominating force in the family to the exclusion and resentment of everyone else. If allowed to, the disabled child can consume an inordinate amount of energy and radically alter the family structure.

In most families the parents do not get their feelings synchronized or are unwilling to share their feelings because they feel they would be imposing. For example, a mother in a parent group spoke about not wanting to tell her husband her fears and anxieties because that just "sets him off." She kept stating "We aren't very good for each other because we pull each other down." The contrary situation is also difficult to deal with: when one parent is heavy in denial while the other parent is deeply distressed. Both parents feel that they lack support from the other and each feels that the spouse just does not understand what is occurring.

Frequently a spouse finds it very hard to listen to and respond to the other's pain. This seems to be especially true of husbands. Men very frequently assign themselves the role of family protector and when some member of their family is in pain that they can do nothing about they feel responsible. This emotion will often trigger a denial reaction. Many men refuse to talk about feelings because it undermines their denial or they invalidate their spouses' feelings by trying to make them feel better. (Professionals tend to do this also.) The inability or unwillingness to talk about feelings between the parents can be very divisive. The professional needs to help the parents resolve the issue around managing each other's grief. The professional needs to be a person whom parents can talk to and cry with without having their feelings invalidated. Often it is desirable to bring both parents together to discuss the dynamics of their relationship around grieving. It is often necessary to try to release the father from the protector role in order to allow him to grieve and to then leave space in their relationship for the wife's grief.

Many changes in the family structure occur when a disabled child is introduced. The husband-wife relationship is altered radically. Wives may have to postpone their careers even further and many economic hardships can occur as a result of the intrusion of the disabled child. Plans are formulated on the availability of schooling and difficult family choices have to be made. Families also lose their privacy or their anonymity when they have a disabled child. For example, parents will often speak about the unsolicited advice and questions they receive from well-meaning strangers when they take their child shopping. (One father solved this problem nicely. When asked by strangers why his young hearing-impaired child was wearing "radios" he would turn to the child and ask him for the score in the baseball game.) Parents need to develop both a thick skin and a sense of humor. Not only is their child different but so are they. They have to put up with the intrusion of strangers and the overheard insensitive comments made by onlookers. One mother commented, "I just can no longer bear taking her shopping with me. I now have to get a babysitter any time I want to go out, and I find that I prefer to stay at home and only see a very limited number of people."

Grandparents. The parents' relationship with their own parents—the child's grandparents—is also altered. The grandparents frequently become fixated in the denial stage, because it is difficult for them to deal with both the pain of having a disabled grandchild and the knowledge that their own child is suffering. The pain comes at a time in life when they are perhaps least prepared to cope with emotional emergencies. The parents, meanwhile, are at the forefront of coping, having to meet with professionals, and are acquiring a sometimes formidable amount of information. Many parents receive some emotional support from either programs or friends and they are able to move through the mourning process much sooner than the grandparents. Very often the parents of the disabled child want to receive succor from their own parents. Unfortunately, what seems to happen in many families is that the parents have to provide support for their own parents.

There is a predictable life crisis in adulthood when we realize that we really do know more than our parents. We then experience the powerful existential feelings of loneliness and responsibility assumption. Having a disabled child accelerates this process, and many parents have to undergo the existential crisis a little sooner than they were prepared for. They often resent the role reversal in their relationship with their own parents, which is brought about by the presence of the disabled child. The parents want so desperately to be parented themselves; instead they find that they are now having to parent their own parents.

To be sure, there are families in which the grandparents assume a dominant role in the rehabilitation process. In those cases they respond much like parents and need a similar time to go through the mourning process. I have found working with grandparents as surrogate parents delightful: they are older and wiser than the other parents in the group and they often bring some needed perspective to the parenting process.

Siblings. At some point, almost all parent groups I have participated in have brought up the problem of siblings. From the parents' perspective, the sibling has to be almost supernormal. The parents have lost all tolerance for the deviant, therefore the normal child carries a heavier burden of the parents' expectations now that they have a disabled child. Parents are often so sensitized to illness and the possibility of disability that they can be overprotective and overanxious with the normal siblings. For example, the younger sibling of a deaf child is probably the child most frequently tested for a hearing disorder. Parents and grandparents are constantly alert to her hearing and not hearing. At the slightest signs of an ear infection the child is rushed to the pediatrician's; speech and language are carefully monitored and any perceived deviation is checked.

Conversely, the siblings receive less positive attention than the disabled child. So much of the parental energy is consumed by the disabled child that the siblings feel less important and often less valued within the family structure. Featherstone (1980) comments:

Meanwhile, brothers and sisters struggle with self-doubt. Some feel apologetic about their own good health, wondering whether they ought to have been stricken instead. Others worry about jealousy: They resent the extra attention paid to the disabled child, but regard their feelings as disloyal and unfair (p. 144).

Older siblings often feel guilty for somehow causing their brother's or sister's disability even though there may be no factual basis for guilt. It also is very difficult for the sibling to express any of the guilt or feelings of anger.

Since no one can turn anger on and off like an electric lamp, many children feel guilty about their rage and resentment, and about the occasions when they vent their frustration on the disabled child himself. The world seems to expect them to love their vulnerable brother or sister with special intensity. They often feel that they do not measure up (Featherstone, 1980, p. 83).

The solutions to the sibling problem are easy to grasp intellectually and very hard to implement practically. Parents need to direct attention to the sibling as a person, not just as a vehicle to help them produce a well-functioning disabled child. Means must be found within the family for the sharing of feelings, and siblings must be given a chance to discuss their feelings of anger and guilt. Unfortunately, the balance is often not easy to achieve as the parents do not have much left for themselves, let alone for the siblings. Parents frequently can identify the problem but, because of limited resources, cannot implement a solution.

THE FAMILY WITH A DISABLED ADULT

The stresses in the family that has a disabled adult are quite similar to those in the family with a disabled child. The stress is related to the strong emotions that are generated by the disability and to the changes in the structure of the family. Malone (1969) interviewed in depth the families of 20 persons with aphasia. He found that the aphasia creates severe problems for the family, which in turn aggravate the condition of the patient. Probably the most pervasive change was the role reversal: wives who were taken care of by their husbands were suddenly themselves caretakers. Husbands who had never assumed any domestic responsibility were now required to do housework in addition to continue being the breadwinner. Children were now required to take care of parents. Families were further stressed by financial problems, health problems, and severe alterations to their social lives. Not surprisingly, these changes generated feelings of guilt and anger. The guilt arose from a feeling that the aphasia was a punishment for a wrong done; the anger was caused by the loss of control.

Kommers and Sullivan (1979), by means of a questionnaire, gathered data from the wives of laryngectomized men. They found problems in health, communication, finances, and occupation. More than 50 percent of the younger wives reported marital changes after the laryngectomy. This study did not provide any interview material, but I think it safe to assume that many of the same difficulties that affected the families of the aphasics would affect the families of laryngectomized patients.

The effects of disability are profound on all members of the family. Families need a great deal of support and help in making the necessary changes. The speech-language pathologist and audiologist are in a key position to help facilitate these changes.

H A B I L I T A T I O N   O F   F A M I L I E S

The literature contains minimal information about the families of catastrophically ill adults and few programs seem to be available. Emerson (1980), after a careful review of the literature on families of aphasics, concludes that "involving the family in rehabilitation is more often stressed in theory than actually practiced." In his study he provided a group experience for the spouses of aphasic patients and found that after group therapy the spouses showed gains in self-esteem and were less depressed compared to a control group, which had had no therapy. Within the spouse group opportunity was provided for the exploration and confirmation of feelings. Bardach (1969) has conducted, in conjunction with a speech therapist, group sessions with wives of aphasic patients. She found that these group sessions were immensely helpful and she, as almost everyone who has written in the field, laments the lack of widespread programs of support for families. Webster (1982), an adult who suffered a cerebrovascular accident, found that "had someone been able to counsel with my family about what to expect from me, their lives would have been much easier."

Alpiner (1978) also found little in the literature about the families of adults with acquired hearing loss. He recommends that the audiologist see the family initially without the hearing-impaired member to give them an understanding of a hearing loss. He then recommends that, if possible, family members attend therapy sessions.

Fleming (1972) has recommended essentially a family counseling approach with hard-of-hearing adults. After a comprehensive audiologic work-up the hearing-impaired person is urged to attend group sessions accompanied by a family member. At these sessions the families get to work out strategies for coping with the hearing impairment. They also get an opportunity to ventilate and share their feelings. For example, in one session I attended, a wife was complaining bitterly about being a "hearing-ear dog" for her husband. By this she meant that she was tired of having to answer the phone, explain the punch lines of jokes, and translate television programs. She received confirmation of her feelings from the other spouses in the group, and she and her husband were able to devise, with the help of the audiologist present, some techniques to improve his hearing. The couple was able to obtain amplifiers for the phone and the television; they were also able to work out some living strategies that would minimize his dependency. In addition, the cathartic experience within the group setting enabled the couple to work constructively on the problem once the interfering feelings had been discharged.

Without weighting this chapter too heavily on the disabled child side, I would like to describe some programmatic options, which we have employed in the Emerson College parent-centered nursery program for deaf children, that involve the families and help reduce the stress. I think that many of these options would be applicable to other family-centered programs with other disabilities.

Habilitating Parents. Unfortunately, most parent education is in practice mother education. This fact generally increases the strain within the marriage as there is a subtle role reversal in the husband-wife relationship. Very often, the wife, by virtue of being actively involved in the educational program, possesses more information and is in a better position to make decisions regarding the child's welfare than is her husband. In some families that have a definite sex-role orientation, the changing role of the wife can be a threat to marital stability. Over the 18-year history of the program, we have seen several marriages founder. I am not sure that the number of failed marriages in this population is any greater than the national statistic on divorce, which is alarming, but it is clear that the deaf child does add more stress to the marriage.

The rational way of attempting to deal with the parent role reversal is to provide more paternal education and support. Fathers seldom receive or solicit emotional support. Almost all support seems to be directed at the mothers. Yet many fathers do need to be listened to and need to be able to talk about their feelings—a fact they may not even realize.

Crowley and colleagues (1982) held a series of bimonthly evening meetings with fathers of the children enrolled in a school for the deaf. During the first year they offered a rather structured content-based program; they then moved into an unstructured group discussion, which encouraged more self-disclosure and feelings. Both fathers and staff concluded that the program was very successful. I suspect that the more structured content-based program may be a good entry point for most fathers. Most men seem to find it difficult to talk about feelings and if some trust and cohesion can develop in the group while they are dealing with structured content, it may be easier for them to subsequently move into affect areas.

Within the Emerson College program we have also tried to involve fathers. We have held nursery on Saturday mornings so that fathers could attend. We have had evening group meetings with fathers only, and we have had husband and wife groups. In the latter groups it was difficult to get much openness, as parents did not want to reveal very much for fear of angering the other spouse. One semester we held a group in which half the men and half the women attended but they were not spouses of each other. This group was a great deal more open (there was a strong confidentiality norm).

Recently we have experimented with intensive weekend experiences without the children. Staff and parents spend 2 days together in a resort setting. Time is set aside for reflection and recreation as well as group meetings. Within this setting, I have used a fishbowl design where one group sits in the center and the rest of the group is silent and on the periphery. The fathers, for example, may talk about how they are affected by their children's deafness while the mothers listen. We then reverse positions, and the mothers talk while the fathers listen. At the end of the session, everybody processes the experience. Other sessions are devoted to large-group discussion. The fishbowl in conjunction with the intensive weekend experience has given us very cohesive parent groups. There has been more subsequent father participation and involvement in all aspects of the program since we initiated the intensive weekend.

Families clearly are changing rapidly. The traditional family, structured along sex-role lines where the mother stays home and takes care of the children and the father is the breadwinner, is rapidly becoming obsolete. We are now seeing many single-parent families and many families in which the wife's income is either principal or absolutely necessary for family survival. Fathers are now generally more involved in direct child-rearing practices, and in several instances, the father has been the family member who has attended the program. These changing roles introduce more stress into the relationships and the parents need a format to work through the problems. A parent-centered program in the discussion-group format can provide them with the means to work through their changing family roles.

I have also found that other families work well (or seem to) with a definite sex-role orientation. I think it important that the communication-disorder professional not impose her values on a family. Direct pressure to try to force father participation should be avoided. In some families this tactic will prove fruitless and may just increase family stress. Fathers can be invited to participate and some programmatic accommodation needs to be made to their life circumstances, such as Saturday or evening meetings. (Several staff members have disputed this, feeling that if it were a medical emergency the father would take time off, therefore, why not for their child's educational program? And so it goes.) If the fathers do not avail themselves of the programmatic options, we must accept their choices.

Habilitating Grandparents. I think that grandparents are generally ignored in most family-centered programs, yet they can and do play a vital role in the health of the family. They can be very supportive of the parents and provide the parents with respite by babysitting the disabled child or providing emotional support. They can also be very draining on the parents' resources by wanting to be taken care of, and by not supporting the parents' habilitative efforts. We have always tried to provide space within the program for grandparents. We generally set aside 1 day for them to come and see their grandchildren in nursery or therapy and to have a group experience with other grandparents. Rarely do grandparents get a chance to meet with other grandparents. From these groups I am always struck by how caring the grandparents are and how little communication there is between generations. Most of the time the grandparents seem to understand more of what is going on than the parents are willing to give them credit for. There seems to be a myth of fragility that impairs parent-grandparent communication. Often parents will not share information with their own parents because "it will just hurt them." Conversely, grandparents do not want to burden their children any further, so there often is minimal communication across generational lines.

On occasion I have used the fishbowl technique of having the grandparents in the center and parents on the periphery, and then reversing positions. For me, it is immensely rewarding to see intergenerational communication take place.

Habilitating Siblings. We have provided a sibling day in our nursery, whereby the deaf child's siblings are invited to participate. Because our program is geared to the very young hearing-impaired child (18 months–3 years) most of the siblings are also young. Depending on their age and understanding, they are made part of the therapy and part of the nursery. Because of their young age I have yet to have a sibling group, something I would dearly love to do. I envision a fishbowl design with siblings, parents, and the disabled children.

The stress on families, which is both a reflection of sociological changes and the change engendered by a disabled person, is not necessarily a negative force. I have seen a great deal of growth occurring as a result of this stress. Many siblings decide to become therapists. While some marriages founder, others are strengthened. For the parents, the disabled child can offer an opportunity to restructure a relationship that has gone stale. Men have often reported how delighted they were to find out how much strength their wives have; the wives were delighted with the caring qualities that emerged from their husbands. Often both parents find a new purpose in working very hard together in parent organizations and therapy programs, and thereby strengthen the bond between them.

Similarly, the parent-grandparent relationship can be restructured. For the first time many parents begin to respond as adults with their own parents and, in time, find themselves being treated as adults. They often begin to see their own parents as vulnerable fellow adults and that is very exciting. For me there has always been growth in stress. I am pushed by stress to develop more capacity in order to reduce the stress. That increased capacity is my growth. I see this happening in all of the families I have worked with, and while I can empathize and perhaps sympathize with the pain involved, I know that if they can just hang in there, they will learn and grow.

There is no doubt in my mind that we can enhance our effectiveness as a profession if we can broaden our scope to include more family work. Unfortunately I think the practice of family work is much like Mark Twain's observation about the weather: people talk about it a great deal but nobody seems to be doing much about it. I think this problem again may be a failure at the training level, and in the next chapter we will look at the training of the student clinician.

BIBLIOGRAPHY

Alpiner, J. Ancillary Personnel in Rehabilitation. In J. Alpiner, *Handbook of Adult Rehabilitative Audiology*. Baltimore: Williams & Wilkins, 1978.

Bardach, J. Group sessions with wives of aphasic patients. *Int. J. Group Psychother.* 19:361, 1969.

Crowley, M., Keane, K., and Needham, C. Fathers: The forgotten parents. *Am. Ann. Deaf* 127:38, 1982.

Edgerly, R. *The Effectiveness of Parent Counseling in the Treatment of Children with Learning Disabilities.* Ph.D. dissertation. Boston University, 1975.

Egolf, D., Shames, G., Johnson, P., and Kasprisin-Burrell, S. The use of parent interaction patterns in therapy for young stutterers. *J. Speech Hear. Disord.* 37:222, 1972.

Elwood, P. C., Johnson, W. R., and Mandeld, J. A. *Parent Centered Programs for Young Hearing Impaired Children.* Maryland: Prince George County Public Schools, 1977.

Emerson, R. *Changes in Depression and Self-esteem of Spouses of Stroke Patients with Aphasia as a Result of Group Counseling.* Ph.D. dissertation. University of Oregon, 1980.

Featherstone, H. *A Difference in the Family.* New York: Basic Books, 1980.

Fleming, M. A total approach to communication therapy. *J. Academy Rehab. Audiology* 5:28, 1972.

Kommers, M. S., and Sullivan, M. D. Wives' evaluation of problems related to laryngectomy. *J. Commun. Disord.* 12:411, 1979.

Malone, R. L. Expressed attitudes of families of aphasics. *J. Speech Hear. Disord.* 34:146, 1969.

Robertson, E., and Suinn, R. The determination of rate of progress of stroke patients through empathy measures of patient and family. *J. Psychosom. Res.* 12:189, 1968.

Satir, V. *Conjoint Family Therapy.* Palo Alto, Calif.: Science and Behavior Books, 1967.

Webster, M. *Hear here.* Newsletter of the Canadian Speech and Hearing Association 6:235, 1982.

CHAPTER 8

EDUCATING THE

STUDENT CLINICIAN

From the humanistic point of view, learning and growth take place best in a nonthreatening atmosphere of warmth and acceptance. In order to accomplish this growth, the therapist needs to be a caring, nonjudgmental, congruent person. None of these skills are exotic; they are within the purview of everyone. The job of the training program is to help develop these attributes in the student clinicians. Unfortunately, almost all graduate training programs tend to stress the intellectual and cognitive skills of the students, and do not emphasize their interpersonal abilities. For example, selection of students is generally on the intellectual skills as exemplified by the Graduate Record Exam scores or grade-point average. Rarely are interpersonal skills considered, except perhaps indirectly as reflected in letters of recommendation. This present era, however, of full disclosure and frequency of litigation, has rendered letters of recommendation almost meaningless. The grade-point average seems to lend an objective measure that we can defend. Interpersonal skills are not readily measurable and are difficult to defend if challenged by an irate student. The danger for our field in not considering interpersonal skills is very great; we can turn out students who are knowledgeable about the field but who are clinically and interpersonally inept.

It would appear, though, that we are selecting reasonably normal graduate students. Crane and Cooper (1983) gave the Minnesota Multiphasic Personality Inventory (MMPI) to 130 female speech-language graduate students. They found that the resultant profiles "were manifestly normal but rather passive, compliant, stereotypically feminine, sensitive, anxious." If this were my profile I might be a bit worried. It concerns me that we are willing to accept these attributes as normal for women. I prefer to think that much of what we are viewing as "stereotypically feminine" is in reality a reflection of our teaching and our attitudes toward women. I hope that this attitude is changing. I am deeply concerned about the passivity and compliance aspects of the personality profile, and what that bodes for our profession. In all fairness Crane and Cooper also found that our students were highly imaginative, creative, and energetic—and I have certainly met and worked with my share of our students with these delightful characteristics. We also know, however, from the research of Miller and Potter (1982) that these students will burn out at an alarming rate.

PROFESSIONAL BURNOUT

The problem of professional burnout in the helping professions is quite severe. Meadow (1981) administered a burnout inventory to 240 teachers of the deaf. Among the findings of her study were:

1. Teachers of the deaf have a higher burnout rate than normal classroom teachers.
2. Burnout is highest among teachers who have been working 7 to 10 years in the job and is lowest among teachers who have been working 11 or more years and among new teachers.
3. Burnout was directly related to perceived ability to influence the work situation. Teachers who felt they had the power to influence their job showed the least burnout.
4. Teachers who showed the highest personal involvement in their jobs also tended to have the highest burnout rate.

The results are I think very interesting. There appears to be a greater stress associated with professionals working with handicapped populations than there is among professionals working with nonhandicapped populations. Young teachers seem to be carried through their first years by idealism and enthusiasm. From the Meadow data and from my own observation, many young beginning teachers get overinvolved with the children. Mattingly (1977) noticed this phenomenon among child-care workers: burnout was signaled by the worker who begins to merge himself and his life with the institution. When this merging occurs the individual loses the resources to give to others. A helping professional is very much like a gasoline station where people come to fill up. At some point though, a truck comes and fills the tanks of the gasoline station. The professional who merges himself with the population he is serving is always among needy people and there is little opportunity to "fill his own tank." I think that this is the professional who burns out within that 7- to 10-year period.

Those professionals who survive beyond the 10-year period of necessity learn better coping strategies. I suspect that they have learned to meet their personal needs outside of their work experiences. I suspect also from the Meadow data that they have a more internal locus of control than do the burnout sufferers. Burnout is directly related to the perceived ability to influence the work situation. Teachers with an inner locus of control are not "pushed into" accepting poor working conditions and are also more likely to assert themselves with administrators.

Within the context and terminologies of this book, burnout can be viewed as primarily a problem in dealing with the existential issue of loneliness and love: the need to be loved can push the teacher into an unwholesome, overinvolved relationship with his students. Burnout can also be seen as an intimacy issue on the Erikson model in that there is a fusion of the personal life and the job. I think overall that burnout is a locus of control problem because people who feel that they have no power, who are like "leaves in the wind," will lose all feeling for their client, will become emotionally exhausted and drained, and will burn out.

I think that we can effect changes in the burnout phenomenon by providing ongoing workshops and inservice for working professionals. I think that a more efficient way of dealing with this problem is by producing students who value themselves, who have an awareness of their own needs, who have an ability to be authentic in relationship, and who have a more internal locus of control and of evaluation.

TRAINING STUDENTS FOR CLINICAL COMPETENCE AND PERSONAL GROWTH

I am not sure that the MMPI measures some of the other important personality variables that will influence clinical competency. The "Annie Sullivan" type of student needs to be identified early in his career. This type is a caring person with a marvelous impulse and energy to be helpful that can be used, but we must provide on the training level experiences to increase self-awareness of his need to be needed. The Annie Sullivan types need to learn how to help in a way that is truly helpful (that is, helping in such a way that the client's self-esteem and independence are not compromised). Our personal satisfactions can come from knowing internally that we have been helpful and not from the approval of others. In short, we also have to develop in students an inner locus of evaluation.

Occasionally we do get interpersonally inept students who are otherwise quite bright, and there needs to be a place within our profession for them. I think they can be helped by some structured interpersonal experiences to become more adept; they may also make good researchers.

Another kind of student occasionally gets through our screening process. This is the student with a very limited capacity to care for others. I think that I can teach almost anything except the capacity to care. This student probably will be a professional disaster despite any technical skills we might teach, and we need to have mechanisms to screen such students out of the profession.

If one examines closely the training of speech pathologists/audiologists, it is apparent that the training is along poorly conceived behavioral lines. Control is generally external to the students. The teacher decides what the students need to know and rewards the students if they appear to learn the material. Student clinicians also learn to please the supervisor, and thus tend to develop an external locus of evaluation. (No wonder they are passive and compliant!) How often do students get a chance to select their own material to be learned, and how often are they required to evaluate themselves and perhaps their supervisor?

During the past several years I have been teaching a course with the wonderfully vague title of "personal dynamics workshop." This is an unstructured course in which the students select the subject matter and are required to grade themselves. The course is very difficult for the students. They are so conditioned to having a curriculum and the expectations of the instructor clearly delineated that they become angry and confused. The anger usually does not surface initially as they do not trust me. It often requires the whole semester just to negotiate the trust issue, and by the time the semester is over, the students are generally ready to get to cognitive material. It is sad to me that the students are so other-directed by virtue of their educational program that they have not learned how to work to satisfy themselves rather than the instructor. I think most of the students who leave the course begin to get a glimmer of what it is like to have an inner locus of control and an inner locus of evaluation.

The communication disorders literature reveals a strong humanistic trend in the supervisory relationship. Ward and Webster (1965) urge that we treat our students as human beings, and think that their self-actualization should be an important consideration in the training program. They argue for courses within the curriculum that are geared to explain human behaviors and which then can be applied to students. Van Riper (1965) delightfully describes the sometimes painful role of the supervisor.

He is a friendly person looking on interested in what is taking place, warmly empathizing with the success and making no issue about the failures. Even when the student is demonstrating outrageous sins of omission or commission the supervisor does not seize the reins. He suffers silently and keeps a pokerface and formulates what he will say to the clinician later (p. 77).

Van Riper believes that we should treat the student clinician with the same loving respect that we wish him to accord the client.

Pickering (1977) argues that the student needs to have skills in relationship as much as knowledge about the field. She believes that the supervisor relationship can be the vehicle for the student to learn about relationships and for promoting personal growth and change in both the supervisor and student clinician; the supervisory relationship needs to have the elements of authenticity, dialogue, risk-taking, and conflict in order to be growth-facilitating.

Caracciolo and colleagues (1978) believe that supervisors should be a role model of the Rogerian, nondirective relationship to the students. The Rogerian relationship would have a high degree of unconditional regard, empathy, and congruence. The students, after experiencing the growth in this humanistic relationship with the supervisor, would then be able to provide this relationship for their clients.

I agree with the premise of Caracciolo and associates that experiencing the humanistic relationship is the best way of learning it. The authors make me uncomfortable, however, when they state later that "it is necessary to define operationally and construct specific training procedures that will develop among supervisors the necessary attitudes and skills that will contribute to personal and professional growth." It seems to me that when we set about "operationally defining" and "developing specific training procedures" we lose the essence of the humanistic approach. At some fundamental level, humanism is ineffable. True learning is an inside-out process, and we must lead students to it and hope they find it by creating the right conditions of a growth-promoting relationship. When we deliberately structure the learning situation so as to teach techniques we are imposing a cognitive solution on an affect problem. Students tend to learn the form of the humanistic approach but not the substance. (Anyone who has tried to have a conversation with a student who thinks that Rogerian reflective listening means repeating back the last thing the person has said begins to get an insight into the causes of homicide.)

Klevans and colleagues (1981) attempted to train students in interpersonal skills. They had two experimental groups; one group was taught skills via extended role playing, having to assume the role of a speech-, language-, or hearing-impaired person in an out-of-class assignment. This was the experiential group. The second group was required to observe clinical interactions and to code behavior. The authors found that the students in the experiential group were able to make significantly more facilitative verbal responses than the coding-observing group when tested in a simulated helping relationship. The authors felt that the total length of time devoted to training (8 3/4 hours) both groups was not sufficient to master interpersonal skills.

I think this study points up several things that need to be examined. If we are going to train students in interpersonal skills, the experience needs to be hands-on rather than didactic. We cannot lecture within a class or even have students observe interactions and then expect them to be interpersonally adept. It is also clear that we have to allot more time within the curriculum for interpersonal skills. The 8 3/4 hours alloted in this study, which was part of a one-credit clinic practice course, is unfortunately typical of most training programs and rather pathetic for attempting to learn such fundamental clinical skills.

I think we also need to attack the problem from the personal growth side. We just cannot limit our endeavors to teaching interpersonal skills from a strictly technical point of view. For me, the best way of teaching and learning counseling has been within the context of my own personal growth experiences. These experiences have included such diverse activities as attendance at workshops, immersion in sensitivity groups, and an Outward Bound learning experience where I had to rock-climb and sail. The latter experience was especially helpful—an underlying theme of that experience was "we have met the enemy and found it is us." I have found that as I have come to accept myself more, I can accept and value others more. I have had to learn to give myself permission to think, to feel, and to be productive.

The dilemma of the supervisor/teaching relationship in developing humanistic relationships with students is the evaluative function held by the teacher. As long as the supervisor/teacher has the power of the grade, locus of control is always external to the student and authenticity on the student's part in relationship to the supervisor is very hard to accomplish. At some level, and at some time, the student must please the teacher in order to get a passing grade. It would require a very high degree of trust to develop authenticity in the relationship, and true equality is not really possible because the situation as far as personal power is concerned is inherently unequal. Van Riper (1965) argues that we should be collaborators with our students rather than supervisors. This ideal is very hard to accomplish because the supervisors must give the students a grade or eventually write a letter of recommendation. While the supervisors may feel that they are collaborators, the students feel differently. It is not surprising that the supervisory relationship looks very different to the student than it does to the supervisor. Culatta and colleagues (1975) found wide discrepancies between the supervisor's and the student clinician's views of their relationship.

In my teaching of content-level courses, I have attempted to work out a compromise between the cognitive and interpersonal learning needs. At the beginning of the course, I give the students the final examination, which consists of a list of essay questions that reflect my opinion as to what content they need to master and from which I will select some unspecified number of questions. I also give the students a bibliography containing readings that will enable them to find the answers to the questions. It is then the student's responsibility to organize his time to master that content. The grade for the course is based solely on the examination performance, and students are encouraged to be as ignorant as possible during class sessions. I usually take responsibility for structuring half of the class sessions with lectures, films, or guest speakers. The students are required to structure the other half of the sessions. The unstructured sessions usually start out with painful silences until the students realize that nothing happens until they make it happen. Periodically we evaluate the class with everyone, including myself, having a chance to talk about how things are going. Within this format, the students get a chance to obtain some control on what they learn, and have to take responsibility for obtaining content. They are never required to read anything. Generally the course evaluations by the students are enthusiastic although whenever we get close to examination time their anxiety begins to increase and they begin to have regrets about their freedom. Because the students are not usually familiar with a learning situation where they have to assume so much responsibility, they frequently have been meeting the demands of other courses and find themselves far behind in our course. Bargaining sessions frequently ensue in which they try to limit the scope of the examination, delay the final, and so on. I delight in the give and take of the negotiations that we engage in, as it reflects an equality and an authenticity in our relationship. I generally remain tough; if the students are to learn responsibility assumption, then they must not be let off the responsibility hook lightly.

My sense of teaching this way is that the students get as much, and often more, content than they did when I took sole responsibility for content. I also am astonished at the interesting byways of content that emerge out of the students' interests. For example, a recent aural rehabilitation class decided to read the play *Children of a Lesser God*, which involves the relationship between a deaf woman and a hearing male speech therapist. From the in-class play reading and discussion, the students obtained a great deal of insight into the problems of deaf-hearing relationships and of contemporary issues among deaf adults. The understanding obtained was of a much deeper dimension than they would have obtained from a review of the didactic literature.

Evidence in the literature suggests that locus of control can be shifted to a more internal orientation as a result of teaching experiences. Johnson and Croft (1975) found that students enrolled in a personalized system of instruction course (PSI) demonstrated a statistically significant shift toward an internal direction as measured by the Rotter scale, after completing the course. The PSI course has no midterms or final examinations; it is entirely self-paced and self-graded. Performance is often evaluated in a personal interview. This sort of course can be modified to become a marvelous blend of behaviorist and humanistic notions. Similarly based courses, which would include more contact with the teacher within a humanistic relationship, could be developed within the field of communication disorders in order to develop self-managing students who also have experienced a clinically and personally useful relationship with a teacher.

In these professionally perilous times of high burnout rate and declining student enrollment, we must find creative solutions to implementing a humanistic-based education, which encourages an inner locus of control. This is not to say that we should give up our cognitive and evaluative functions; we must supplement content with interpersonal learning. It is unreasonable to expect students trained within the current poorly conceived behavioral model to easily take responsibility for themselves and for the profession. The behavioral model, with its emphasis on external locus of control and external locus of evaluation, will tend to produce professionals who will accept poor working conditions, who will work mechanically, and who will not take responsibility for furthering the profession—by passively and compliantly accepting things as they are. If we do not anticipate change and act, we will be overwhelmed by it. The future of our profession, I think, rests in altering our current educational practices to include a more humanistic base, which will in turn create a more self-confident, self-reliant, and assertive professional, a professional who will also be much more effective in serving the communicatively disordered. We owe our clients and our profession no less.

BIBLIOGRAPHY

Caracciolo, G., Rigrodsky, S., and Morrison, E. A Rogerian orientation to the speech-language pathology supervisory relationship. *ASHA* 20:286, 1978.

Crane, S., and Cooper, E. Speech-language clinician personality variables and clinical effectiveness. *J. Speech Hear. Disord.* 48:140, 1983.

Culatta, R., Colucci, S., and Wiggins, E. Clinical supervisors and trainees: Two views of a process. *ASHA* 17:152, 1975.

Johnson, W., and Croft, R. Locus of control and participation in a personalized system of instruction course. *J. Educ. Psychol.* 67:416, 1975.

Klevans, D., Volz, H., and Friedman, R. A comparison of experimental and observational approaches for enhancing the interpersonal communication skills of speech-language pathology students. *J. Speech Hear. Disord.* 46:208, 1981.

Mattingly, M. A. Sources of stress and burn-out in professional child care work. *Child Care Quarterly* 6:127, 1977.

Meadow, K. Burnout in professionals working with deaf children. *Am. Ann. Deaf* 126:13, 1981.

Miller, M., and Potter, R. Professional burnout among speech-language pathologists. *ASHA* 24:177, 1982.

Pickering, M. An examination of concepts operative in the supervisory process and relationship. *ASHA* 19:697, 1977.

Van Riper, C. Supervision of clinical practice. *ASHA* 7:75, 1965.

Ward, B., and Webster, E. The training of clinical personnel. II. A concept of clinical preparation. *ASHA* 7:103, 1965.

INDEX